SBAs and EMQs in Surgery for Medical Students

ANNA KOWALEWSKI

Foundation Doctor

Charing Cross Hospital, London, UK

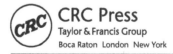

CRC Press
Taylor & Francis Group
Boca Raton London New York

CRC Press is an imprint of the
Taylor & Francis Group, an **informa** business

Anna Kowalewski has asserted her right under the Copyright, Designs and Patents Act 1988 to be identified as the author of this work.

First published 2014 by Radcliffe Publishing

Published 2021 by CRC Press
Taylor & Francis Group
6000 Broken Sound Parkway NW, Suite 300
Boca Raton, FL 33487-2742

© 2014 by Taylor & Francis Group, LLC
CRC Press is an imprint of Taylor & Francis Group, an Informa business

No claim to original U.S. Government works

ISBN-13: 978-1-84619-466-5 (pbk)

Visit the Taylor & Francis Web site at
http://www.taylorandfrancis.com

and the CRC Press Web site at
http://www.crcpress.com

British Library Cataloguing in Publication Data

A catalogue record for this book is available from the British Library.

Typeset by Darkriver Design, Auckland, New Zealand

Contents

Preface   v

About the author   vi

Single best answer questions   1

  1 Gastroenterology   3

     Answers   12

  2 Hepatobiliary   17

     Answers   24

  3 Breast   27

     Answers   34

  4 Vascular   37

     Answers   44

  5 Hernias   47

     Answers   54

  6 Urology   57

     Answers   64

  7 Orthopaedics   67

     Answers   74

  8 Ear, nose and throat   77

     Answers   81

9   Neck   83
    Answers   87

10 Trauma   89
    Answers   99

Extended matching questions   **103**
    Questions 1–20   105
    Answers 1–20   127

Index   151

Preface

This is the surgical SBA and EMQ book to end all others. Use this book to inform your learning. Use it as a starting point or at the end of your revision to see what you need to learn or test what you know – invaluable. This comprehensive guide tests your knowledge of multiple specialties including upper and lower gastrointestinal surgery, vascular surgery, urology, orthopaedics and trauma, and breast and neck surgery. It helps you understand the concepts rather than just learning the facts.

The book contains 190 single best answer questions and 100 extended matching questions, with varying complexity to test your knowledge and highlight any deficiencies in your learning. These range from important questions explaining basic concepts to interesting questions that will help develop your clinical knowledge in an organic way. Furthermore, crucially, the answers are explained in a full and comprehensive way. Each answer includes helpful hints and tips to aid your learning and continuing education, both in exams and in your future career.

Anna Kowalewski
September 2013

About the author

Anna Kowalewski graduated from Imperial College London having gained a first for her Bachelor of Science (Honours) degree and a distinction in her finals. During her undergraduate years, Anna was awarded the Medical Student Prize from the Royal College of Paediatrics and Child Health and the John Adamson Prize in Paediatrics, along with a number of other distinctions. She started her training at Imperial College Healthcare NHS Trust. A keen advocate for medical student education, Anna keenly believes in lighting a fire rather than filling the pail.

Single best answer questions

Gastroenterology

Q1 A 60-year-old woman presents with difficulty in swallowing. On examination you note she has koilonychia and angular stomatitis. She denies any weight loss. Which is the most likely diagnosis?

a Crohn's disease

b Plummer–Vinson syndrome

c Oesophagitis

d Oesophageal varices

e Oesophageal malignancy

Q2 A 47-year-old patient is to undergo a Heller's cardiomyotomy operation. What is the most likely diagnosis?

a Plummer–Vinson syndrome

b Carcinoma of the oesophagus

c Achalasia

d Atresia of the oesophagus

e Oesophagitis

Q3 A 63-year-old male patient has been diagnosed with oesophageal squamous cell carcinoma. What is the most likely aetiological cause for this condition?

a Alcohol

b Achalasia

c Nitrosamines

d High-salt diet

e Vitamin C deficiency

Q4 You are a general practitioner and a 64-year-old male presents with new-onset dyspepsia. What is the next most appropriate step in management?

a Advise change in diet

b Prescribe proton pump inhibitor and review in 1 month

c Review medications for possible causes of dyspepsia

d Routine referral for endoscopy

e Urgent referral for endoscopy

Q5 Which of the following statements about Mallory–Weiss tears is not true?

a They usually present after an episode of vomiting

b It is a longitudinal tear in the oesophagus

c They are inevitably fatal

d There is an increased risk of developing the tear in those who are alcohol dependent

e None of the above

Q6 A 45-year-old male patient is noted to have Barrett's oesophagus. Which one of the following cell changes occurs in Barrett's oesophagus?

a Dysplasia

b Anaplasia

c Hyperplasia

d Metaplasia

e Neoplasia

Q7 Which of the following will most likely be used to replace the oesophagus in cases where extensive oesophagectomy is undertaken?

a Jejunum

b Ileum

c Transverse colon

d Descending colon

e Rectum

Q8 The following are all well-recognised complications of Crohn's disease **except**?

a Erythema multiforme

b Iritis

c Anal fistulae

d Polyarthropathy

e Megaloblastic anaemia

Q9 A 70-year-old patient presents with a recent change in bowel habit, absolute constipation and abdominal distension. Which investigation is most likely to lead to a diagnosis?

a Routine bloods including C-reactive protein, full blood count and urea and electrolytes

b Plain supine abdominal radiograph

c Barium swallow

d Barium meal

e Proctoscopy

Q10 A 63-year-old man presents with dysphagia. He explains that he first had trouble swallowing solids but now has trouble swallowing liquids too. The following are all appropriate steps in the development of a management plan **except?**

a Barium/Gastrografin swallow

b Chest radiograph

c Routine bloods including liver function tests

d Total parenteral nutrition

e Upper gastrointestinal endoscopy with or without biopsy

Q11 A 37-year-old female presents with nausea, vomiting, abdominal pain and distension. She has a past medical history of ulcerative colitis. Which investigation is most likely to lead to a diagnosis?

a Routine bloods including full blood count, liver function tests and C-reactive protein

b Plain abdominal radiograph

c Abdominal ultrasound scan

d Colonoscopy

e MRI of the abdomen

Q12 An 86-year-old woman presents with dysphagia. She explains that she often 'brings her solid food up'. You note she is suffering from halitosis despite relatively good oral care. On examination there is a small lump present on the left side of her neck. Which investigation is most likely to lead to a diagnosis?

a   Barium swallow

b   Endoscopy

c   Neck radiograph

d   Neck ultrasound scan

e   Referral to ear, nose and throat

Q13 Following a recent day admission for the removal of a fish bone from her oesophagus via rigid oesophagoscopy, a 62-year-old lady presents with severe chest pain. She is thought to be suffering from an oesophageal perforation. Which investigation is most likely to lead to a diagnosis?

a   Barium swallow

b   Endoscopy

c   Gastrografin swallow

d   Soft tissue plain radiograph of the neck

e   Upright plain chest radiograph

Q14 A 61-year-old patient presents with central colicky abdominal pain that lasts for a few minutes. She has also been vomiting. She is not constipated. On examination you note multiple scars on her abdomen and generalised abdominal distension. What is the most likely aetiological cause?

a   Adhesions

b   Crohn's disease

c   Gallstone ileus

d   Hernia

e   Neoplasm

Q15 A 61-year-old patient presents with lower abdominal pain. She reports no vomiting but thinks she has not passed flatus or faeces for 24 hours. On examination her abdomen is hyper-resonant and has developed generalised abdominal distension. What is the most likely aetiological cause?

a Adhesions

b Colonic atresia

c Crohn's disease

d Hernia

e Neoplasm

Q16 An otherwise healthy 64-year-old presents with recent-onset abdominal pain and alteration in bowel habit. She undergoes a left hemicolectomy. What is the most likely diagnosis?

a Caecal carcinoma

b Carcinoma located at the transverse colon

c Carcinoma located at the splenic flexure

d Sigmoid carcinoma

e Rectal carcinoma

Q17 A 6-month-old baby presents with her mother. Her mother states that she has found mucus and blood in the nappy. The baby screams and appears to have abdominal pain, although she seems fine and settles between these episodes. The mother also notes her child has recently commenced eating solid food. What is the most likely diagnosis?

a Anal fissure

b Gastroenteritis

c Intussusception

d Meckel's diverticulum

e Volvulus

Q18 A 57-year-old woman presents with dysphagia. On examination you note she has koilonychia and angular stomatitis. She denies any weight loss. Which management plan would you instigate first?

a Iron replacement therapy alone

b Iron replacement therapy and balloon dilatation

c Endoscopic banding

d Further investigations to establish staging of tumour

e No treatment is required

Q19 Which of the following is not a classical symptom for the presentation of intestinal obstruction?

a Abdominal distension

b Absolute constipation

c Colicky pain

d Melaena

e Vomiting

Q20 A 6-week-old baby presents with his mother. The child presents with dehydration due to projectile vomiting after feeding. The baby is hungry. On examination a palpable mass can be felt in the right upper quadrant. Which is the most appropriate management plan?

a No treatment required

b Duodenostomy

c Exploratory laparotomy

d Hydrostatic reduction by barium enema

e Ramstedt's pyloromyotomy

Q21 A patient undergoes a restorative proctocolectomy. What is the most likely diagnosis?

a Crohn's disease

b Tubular adenoma

c Rectal carcinoma

d Ulcerative colitis

e Volvulus

Q22 A 41-year-old male is found to suffer from rectal carcinoma. What is the most likely aetiological cause for his neoplasia?

a Alcohol

b Smoking

c Diet

d Previous irradiation

e Adenomatous polyposis coli (APC) mutation on chromosome 5

Q23 Most colorectal tumours are resected simply at the tumour borders. However, one tumour also often involves the mesentery and thus necessitates its removal. What is the most likely diagnosis?

a Right-sided colonic tumour

b Transverse colonic tumour

c Left-sided colonic tumour

d Sigmoid tumour

e Rectal tumour

Q24 A 57-year-old female presents with a fever, vomiting and severe left lower abdominal pain. On examination you note she has rebound tenderness and guarding in the left iliac fossa. What is the next most appropriate step in management?

a Intravenous broad-spectrum antibiotics

b Rigid sigmoidoscopy

c Resection and primary anastomosis

d Proximal loop colostomy

e Hartmann's procedure

Q25 A 47-year-old complains of chest pain, which wakes him in the early hours of the morning. He drinks 21 units a week and smokes 40 cigarettes a day. He finds food lessens the pain. He is currently taking no medication. What is the most likely diagnosis?

a Angina

b Costochondritis

c Duodenal ulcer

d Gastric ulcer

e Oesophagitis

Answers

A₁   b

This patient has developed Plummer–Vinson syndrome, the formation of an oesophageal web (above the level of the aortic arch) in association with iron deficiency anaemia.

A₂   c

This patient is suffering from achalasia, which is the failure of the lower oesophageal sphincter to relax. This is often in association with a degeneration of Auerbach's plexus. Heller's cardiomyotomy involves complete division of the circular muscle at the level of the oesophagogastric junction. Note there has been a recent move to laparoscopic minimal access surgery for the condition.

A₃   a

Alcohol and smoking are the most common causes of oesophageal cancer. The others included are less common causes but may still be contributing factors. Note that 90% are squamous cell carcinomas and thus occur in the upper two-thirds of the oesophagus.

A₄   e

As per National Institute for Health and Care Excellence guidelines, new-onset dyspepsia in a patient aged 55 years or over should be treated as carcinoma (most likely gastric) until proven otherwise. Up to 2% of dyspeptic cases may be found to have gastric carcinoma at endoscopy.

A₅   c

Bleeding usually stops spontaneously after 24–48 hours. If treatment is required, cauterisation or injection of adrenaline to the artery may be undertaken during endoscopy. Very rarely, embolisation of the artery supplying the region may be required.

A6 d

Barrett's oesophagus is the abnormal metaplastic change in the lower end of the oesophagus thought to be due to chronic acid reflux. The normal squamous epithelium is replaced by columnar epithelium (intestinal-like). It confers an increased risk of adenocarcinoma.

A7 c

The transverse colon is used, as it is easily mobilised, has a good blood supply and will not stenose as small bowel will.

A8 a

Erythema multiforme is an acute, self-limiting hypersensitivity skin reaction caused by infections and medications. The lesions are described as target lesions. Target lesions are circular with a central blister. In Crohn's disease, the patient is most likely to suffer from erythema nodosum, which is an inflammation of the fat under the skin (panniculitis). It manifests itself as red nodules, most often over the patient's shins.

A9 b

A plain supine abdominal radiograph will show dilated loops of large bowel, indicating a large bowel obstruction. Note, it is obviously important to record routine bloods, but this will not lead to a diagnosis. In patients where the symptoms are equivocal, a CT scan or contrast enema may be employed to confirm the diagnosis.

A10 d

Total parenteral nutrition would not be used in this patient, as it would seem the problem is located in the oesophagus and there is no apparent problem with digestion, only conduction of nutrients. The patient could be fed through a nasogastric tube or, if required, by percutaneous endoscopic gastrostomy.

A11 b

This patient has a history of ulcerative colitis, which gives her an increased risk of developing toxic megacolon. This would be seen with a plain abdominal radiograph and would be shown by major dilatation of the entire colon. Such dilatation puts the colon at risk of perforation. While dilated bowel loops may be seen by other modalities, a supine abdominal radiograph is quick, has minimal risk and is accurate in these cases.

A₁₂ a

This patient has a Zenker's diverticulum, a diverticulum of the mucosa of the pharynx (about the cricopharyngeal muscle). Consequently, the most beneficial investigation is a barium swallow. If the diverticulum is small and asymptomatic it may be treated conservatively. However, if the diverticulum is larger it may be resected by either open or endoscopic surgery.

A₁₃ c

It may be possible to observe air in the soft tissue on plain radiographs. However, the leaked air may be small in volume and consequently a Gastrografin swallow is able to determine whether there is indeed a perforation and the site at which the perforation has occurred. A barium swallow is contraindicated, as barium sulphate is an irritant outside the gastrointestinal tract.

A₁₄ a

This patient appears to be suffering from a small bowel obstruction. Apart from in a virgin abdomen (an abdomen that has not been operated upon), the most common cause of a small bowel obstruction is adhesions.

A₁₅ e

Neoplasia is the most common cause of large bowel obstruction. Therefore, in contrast to most causes of small bowel obstruction, they will nearly all be operated upon. The others may all cause large bowel obstruction. The most common causes after neoplasia are volvulus (often sigmoid), hernia diverticulitis and inflammatory bowel disease.

A₁₆ c

This patient is suffering from carcinoma located at the splenic flexure. Forty per cent of cancers present as a surgical emergency with either obstruction or perforation. Emergency presentation is associated with a poorer outcome.

A₁₇ c

Intussusception is where one part of the bowel invaginates into an adjacent part. The peak incidence occurs between 6 and 9 months of age. It can, however, be caused by a Meckel's diverticulum. Classically, it presents with intermittent colicky pain and vomiting, with each episode lasting for 2 minutes every 20 minutes. Reduction can be attempted with air or contrast enema under radiological guidance. If a patient is in shock they will require surgery and maybe even bowel resection.

A₁₈ b

This patient has developed Plummer–Vinson syndrome, the formation of an oesophageal web (above the level of the aortic arch) in association with iron deficiency anaemia. The most appropriate management plan in this case is iron replacement with balloon dilatation. The balloon dilatation will be undertaken through endoscopy.

A₁₉ d

Melaena is the passage of black tarry stools caused by the presence of altered blood. This bleeding occurs above the level of the ileo-caecal valve and equates to more than 60 mL of blood loss. Even if a patient's obstruction is causing some bleeding, the patient will usually not suffer from melaena due to absolute constipation.

A₂₀ e

The child has pyloric stenosis (usually confirmed by history and ultrasound). The patient may be suffering from electrolyte imbalance due to repeated vomiting. This should be corrected prior to any surgery. Ramstedt's pyloromyotomy is a longitudinal incision in the pylorus down to the mucosa.

A₂₁ d

The patient is most likely to have ulcerative colitis. If the patient presents as an emergency he or she will most likely have a total colectomy with ileostomy and mucus fistula. However, if the procedure is elective, the most effective treatment is a restorative proctocolectomy with an ileal pouch. This gives the patient better functional results.

A22 e

In this case the patient is young. Consequently, it is likely the patient has inherited a predisposition to the formation of multiple polyps and the increased risk of developing colorectal cancer. Apart from alcohol, all the other factors cause an increased risk of colorectal cancer.

A23 e

It is important to understand that most rectal tumours spread radially and thus involve the mesentery. This total mesorectal excision takes place during an anterior resection to ensure removal of the entire tumour.

A24 e

This patient is most likely suffering from an acute diverticulum perforation with associated signs of peritonitis. The segment of bowel affected must be resected (subtotal colectomy) with the formation of a proximal colostomy (or ileostomy) and the oversewing of the rectal stump. Note that although this is a reversal operation, up to two-thirds never have the reversal.

A25 c

This is the classic description of a duodenal ulcer.

2

Hepatobiliary

Q₁ The following are all associated with the development of acute pancreatitis **except**?

a Gallstones

b Alcohol

c Diabetes mellitus

d Corticosteroids

e Hyperlipidaemia

Q₂ A 47-year-old homeless man presents with haematemesis. He smells strongly of alcohol. His blood pressure is 95/60 and pulse is 100. What is the next most appropriate step in management?

a Oxygen and intravenous fluids

b Contrast swallow

c Endoscopy

d Chest radiograph

e Blood tests

Q3 A 37-year-old females presents with severe epigastric pain radiating to her back. Of note, she recently commenced a regimen of high-dose steroids and azathioprine for an exacerbation of Crohn's. What is the most likely diagnosis?

a Acute pancreatitis

b Ischaemic bowel

c Perforated peptic ulcer

d Small bowel obstruction

e Toxic megacolon

Q4 Courvoisier's law states: 'in the presence of a palpable gallbladder, painless jaundice is . . .' The following are all incorrect **except**?

a Is likely to be caused by gallstones

b Is unlikely to be caused by gallstones

c Is never due to malignancy

d Is likely due to carcinoma of the tail of the pancreas

e Is likely due to carcinoma of the head of the pancreas

Q5 A 43-year-old female presents with a 24-hour history of constant pain in her right side. On examination she is tender in the right upper quadrant and you are able to elicit Murphy's sign. What is the next most appropriate initial investigation?

a Abdominal radiograph

b Endoscopy

c Endoscopic retrograde cholangiopancreatography

d Serum bilirubin

e Ultrasound scan of the abdomen

Q6 What is the next most appropriate step in management of the patient from the previous question?

a Conservative with intravenous fluids

b Oral antibiotics

c Endoscopic retrograde cholangiopancreatography

d Laparoscopic cholecystectomy

e Open cholecystectomy

Q7 A 57-year-old woman is diagnosed with pancreatic cancer. Further investigations reveal the cancer is located in the head of the pancreas. Of the following, which is the appropriate treatment?

a Chemotherapy

b Chemotherapy and radiotherapy

c Distal pancreatectomy

d Total pancreatectomy

e Whipple's procedure (pancreaticoduodenectomy)

Q8 A 47-year-old woman presents with vomiting, a low-grade fever and upper abdominal pain. On examination you note she is obese but can still palpate a small tender mass in her right upper quadrant. There are no other signs. What is the most likely diagnosis?

a Acute cholecystitis

b Biliary colic

c Cholangitis

d Gastroenteritis

e Gastric ulcer

Q9 A patient returns to your firm 4 weeks post cholecystectomy with jaundice. He has also noticed his urine is dark but his stools are pale. What is the most likely diagnosis?

a Acute cholecystitis

b Chronic cholecystitis

c Carcinoma of the head of the pancreas

d Primary biliary cirrhosis

e Stone in the common bile duct

Q10 Initial investigations for jaundice include all of the following **except?**

a Abdominal radiograph

b Endoscopic retrograde cholangiopancreatography

c Liver function tests

d Clotting function

e Hepatitis virology

Q11 Complications of high-dose steroid therapy include all of the following **except?**

a Acute pancreatitis

b Diabetes mellitus

c Peptic ulceration

d Osteoporosis

e Weight loss

Q12 Complications of acute cholecystitis include all of the following **except?**

a Gangrenous cholecystitis

b Gallstone ileus

c Gallbladder perforation

d Cholecystoenteric fistula

e Gallbladder carcinoma

Q13 A patient returns after cholecystectomy with jaundice and painful right-sided abdominal spasms and is found to have retained common bile duct stones. What is the next most appropriate step in management?

    a Direct endoscopic removal

    b Endoscopic retrograde cholangiopancreatography and sphincterotomy

    c Laser lithotripsy

    d Surgical exploration

    e Conservative treatment

Q14 A 43-year-old female undergoes a routine laparoscopic cholecystectomy that converts to an open procedure on the operating table because of difficulty in mobilising the gallbladder. Her recovery is slow and on the third operative day she starts to develop a fever that spikes cyclically over the next 2 days. Her chest radiograph is normal and her bloods show a raised white cell count but are otherwise normal. What is the next most appropriate initial investigation?

    a Abdominal radiograph

    b Conservative, no further investigation required

    c Immediate return to surgery for laparotomy

    d CT scan of the abdomen

    e Ultrasound scan of the abdomen

Q15 The following are all associated with ascending cholangitis **except**?

    a Carcinoma of the head of the pancreas

    b Gallstones

    c Cholangiocarcinoma

    d Large bowel obstruction

    e Benign stricture of the common bile duct

Q16 The following are all associated with the investigation of jaundice **except**?

   a Abdominal radiograph will show gallstones in up to 90% of cases

   b Chest radiograph may show raised right diaphragm

   c Full blood count showing anaemia

   d Raised serum transaminases

   e Prolonged prothrombin time

Q17 It is 3.30 a.m. on a Sunday morning and a 38-year-old alcohol-dependent man presents with massive haematemesis. After immediate resuscitation you have established central venous access and he is receiving O negative blood. Type-specific blood is on its way. However, the bleeding has not stopped. There is no endoscopist available. What is the next most appropriate step in management?

   a Wait for type-specific blood

   b Wait for an available endoscopist

   c Insert a Sengstaken–Blakemore tube

   d Start neomycin

   e Start lactulose

Q18 A 17-year-old girl presents with right lower abdomen pain and associated nausea and vomiting. She has no past medical history of note. On examination she is acutely tender in the right iliac fossa. The following are all possible diagnoses **except**?

   a Appendicitis

   b Diverticulitis

   c Ectopic pregnancy

   d Gastroenteritis

   e Torsion of ovarian cyst

Q19 What is the most likely infective aetiological cause of cholangiocarcinoma?

a *Clonorchis sinensis*

b *Escherichia coli*

c *Enterococcus*

d *Klebsiella*

e *Pseudomonas*

Q20 Common complications after laparoscopic cholecystectomy include all of the following **except**?

a Bleeding

b Jaundice

c Infection

d Paralytic ileus

e Retained stone in the bile duct

Answers

A1 c
Remember the mnemonic I GET SMASHED. Idiopathic, Gallstones, Ethanol, Trauma, Steroids, Mumps (and other viruses), Autoimmune disease (e.g. systemic lupus erythematosus), Scorpion (*Tityus trinitatis*) stings, Hypercalcaemia (hyperlipidaemia), Endoscopic retrograde cholangiopancreatography, Drugs.

A2 a
Remember ABC – airway, breathing and circulation. This man requires resuscitation. After he is made stable he can go to the endoscopy suite. He is most likely suffering from varices.

A3 a
Remember the mnemonic I GET SMASHED. Idiopathic, Gallstones, Ethanol, Trauma, Steroids, Mumps (and other viruses), Autoimmune disease (e.g. systemic lupus erythematosus), Scorpion (*Tityus trinitatis*) stings, Hypercalcaemia (hyperlipidaemia), Endoscopic retrograde cholangiopancreatography, Drugs (including azathioprine).

A4 b
While painless jaundice with a palpable gallbladder may be due to pancreatic malignancy, the law states it is unlikely to be caused by gallstones – gallstones being a chronic condition leading to a fibrotic and small gallbladder.

A5 e
Ultrasound scan is the initial investigation of choice. Diagnostic features include presence of gallstones and a distended, thick-walled gallbladder. Remember Murphy's sign, guarding in right upper quadrant on deep inspiration.

A6 a

Eighty per cent of patients improve with conservative treatment.

A7 e

Resection is necessary for cure, yet only 15% of tumours are thought to be resectable. The head of the pancreas and duodenum is excised. Then end-to-side pancreaticojejunostomy, end-to-side hepaticojejunostomy and duodenojejunostomy.

A8 a

This patient is suffering from acute cholecystitis. Fever and right upper quadrant pain are typical. Vomiting and nausea are often mentioned as part of the history. The patient may mention that pain occurs after fatty meals. Murphy's sign may be present. Note, while Murphy's sign has a high sensitivity the specificity is not high. Also note in the elderly the sensitivity is much lower.

A9 e

The most common cause of extrahepatic cholestasis is gallstones in the bile duct.

A10 b

Endoscopic retrograde cholangiopancreatography is not an initial investigation for jaundice. Obviously, it may come later.

A11 e

Patients will usually experience weight gain.

A12 e

While gallbladder carcinoma is a complication of chronic cholecystitis, the others are all complications of acute cholecystitis.

A13 b

The most appropriate treatment is for the patient to undergo endoscopic retrograde cholangiopancreatography and sphincterotomy. It will allow the stone to pass and also allow future stones to pass.

A₁₄ e

The patient is likely to be suffering from an abscess, which can be identified by ultrasound.

A₁₅ d

Large bowel obstructions do not affect the hepatobiliary system and are unlikely to cause ascending cholangitis.

A₁₆ a

An abdominal radiograph will show gallstones in only 10% of cases.

A₁₇ c

In the case of an upper gastrointestinal haemorrhage where endoscopy cannot be performed, a Sengstaken–Blakemore tube may be inserted as a temporary measure until the patient is stable and an endoscopy can be performed. While neomycin and lactulose may be helpful post cessation of bleeding, they are not helpful in extremis.

A₁₈ b

While diverticulitis may be a possibility in an elderly patient, it is unlikely in a young patient with no past medical history.

A₁₉ a

Clonorchis sinensis is a liver fluke that is localised to the gallbladder and can lead to cholangiocarcinoma. The others may cause cholecystitis.

A₂₀ d

Patients who undergo laparoscopic treatment tend to have quicker returns to full activity. Paralytic ileus is the functional obstruction commonly seen after major abdominal open surgery.

3

Breast

Q1 The following are all possible signs of carcinoma of the breast **except?**

a Peau d'orange

b Wedge fracture of the vertebral column

c Inversion of the nipple

d Nipple discharge

e Cervical lymphadenopathy

Q2 The following are all possible signs of fibroadenoma of the breast **except?**

a Cyclical pain

b Usually presents with multiple lumps

c The lump is highly mobile

d Most common in women in their second or third decade

e Composed of fibrous and glandular tissue

Q3 The following are all risk factors for breast carcinoma **except?**

a Presence of ductal carcinoma in situ

b Family history

c Smoking

d Obesity

e Alcohol

Q4 A 28-year-old woman presents with a left breast lump. On examination she has a 1 × 1 × 1 cm breast lump. What is the next most appropriate step in management?

a Excisional biopsy

b Fine needle aspiration

c Mammogram

d Core biopsy

e Ultrasound scan of the breasts

Q5 A 53-year-old male presents with gynaecomastia. He denies any recreational drug use, although he does take tablets, which he thinks are for his blood pressure. What is the most likely aetiological factor for his gynaecomastia?

a Drugs

b Persistent pubertal gynaecomastia

c Cirrhosis

d Primary hypogonadism

e Testicular tumour

Q6 The following facts are correct about ductal carcinoma in situ **except?**

a It is a premalignant condition

b It does not confer an increased risk of invasive breast carcinoma

c It may present with an isolated breast lump

d It is often identified through mammography

e It does not produce a nipple discharge

Q7 Which of the following is the most common site affected by breast cancer

a Upper inner quadrant

b Upper outer quadrant

c Lower inner quadrant

d Lower outer quadrant

e Retro-areolar

Q8 A 63-year-old woman presents with a breast lump. Which management plan would you instigate first?

a Clinical examination and mammogram

b Clinical examination, ultrasound scan and biopsy

c Ultrasound scan, mammogram and biopsy

d Clinical examination, mammogram and biopsy

e Clinical examination, chest radiograph and biopsy

Q9 A 34-year-old woman presented with a painful breast. On examination you note there is nipple retraction and nipple discharge. The breast ducts are not dilated. What is the most likely diagnosis?

a Periductal mastitis

b Duct ectasia

c Fat necrosis

d Duct papilloma

e Fibroadenoma

Q10 A 34-year-old woman presented with a painful breast. On examination you note there is nipple retraction and nipple discharge. What is the next most appropriate step in management?

a Reassurance

b Analgesia

c Analgesia and antibiotics

d Evening primrose oil tablets

e Urgent referral to breast clinic

Q11 A 27-year-old woman presents with nipple discharge and bleeding. On examination you note she has a painful subareolar nodule in her left breast and also multiple lumps in her left breast. What is the most likely diagnosis?

a Periductal mastitis

b Duct ectasia

c Fat necrosis

d Duct papilloma

e Fibroadenoma

Q12 A 27-year-old woman presents with nipple discharge and bleeding. On examination you note she has a painful subareolar nodule in her left breast and also multiple lumps in her left breast. What is the next most appropriate step in management?

a Reassurance

b Analgesia

c Antibiotics

d Analgesia and antibiotics

e Urgent referral to breast clinic and mammography

Q13 A 62-year-old woman presents with a lump in her breast. On examination you note the lump is almost 3 cm in diameter. Biopsy reveals the patient is suffering from invasive ductal carcinoma. The following are all first-line investigations for the staging of breast carcinoma **except**?

a Full blood count

b Chest radiograph

c Liver ultrasound scan

d Liver function tests

e Erythrocyte sedimentation rate

Q14 A 62-year-old woman presents with a lump in her breast. On examination you note the lump is almost 2 cm in diameter. Biopsy reveals the patient is suffering from invasive ductal carcinoma. The following are all viable treatment options for cure **except?**

a Wide local excision

b Wide local excision with radiotherapy

c Wide local excision with radiotherapy and chemotherapy

d Mastectomy

e Mastectomy and chemotherapy

Q15 A 67-year-old woman underwent a radical mastectomy 10 years ago. She is now experiencing complications from her operation and adjuvant therapy. The following are all complications from radical mastectomy and its adjuvant therapy **except?**

a Lymphoedema

b Difficulty in psychological adjustment

c Sarcoma

d Intercostal brachial nerve numbness

e Haematoma

Q16 A 74-year-old woman presented with a painful breast. On examination you note there is nipple retraction and nipple discharge is cheesy. There are no palpable lumps. What is the most likely diagnosis?

a Periductal mastitis

b Duct ectasia

c Fat necrosis

d Duct papilloma

e Fibroadenoma

Q17 A 74-year-old woman presented with a painful breast. On examination you note there is nipple retraction and nipple discharge is cheesy. There are no palpable lumps. She is not bothered by the condition usually, but her daughter urged her to see the doctor. What is the next most appropriate step in management?

a Reassurance

b Simple analgesia

c Antibiotics and simple analgesia

d Excision

e Mastectomy

Q18 A 72-year-old woman presents to her general practitioner with a lump in her breast. It had not been causing her any pain or discomfort, although it has been growing in size over the past 18 months. On examination you note the lump is almost 6 cm in diameter, is causing skin tethering and in-drawing of the nipple. What is the most likely diagnosis?

a Breast abscess

b Breast cyst

c Breast carcinoma

d Ductal carcinoma in situ

e Fat necrosis

Q19 A 39-year-old woman presents with a breast lump. The history is unclear, but on examination you note that she has large breasts and the lump is fixed to the skin and not deep structures. What is the most likely diagnosis?

a Fat necrosis

b Fibroadenoma

c Intraductal papilloma

d Microcalcifications

e Simple cyst

Q20 A 56-year-old female presents after a routine mammogram found diffuse microcalcifications. What is the next most appropriate step in management?

a Fine needle aspiration

b Stereotactic core needle biopsy

c Repeat mammogram

d Repeat mammogram in 1 year

e Ultrasound scan of the breast

Answers

A₁ e

The breast drains to the maxillary lymph nodes. All the other signs may be signs of breast carcinoma.

A₂ b

Fibroadenoma occasionally presents as multiple lumps but usually as a single, discrete, firm, non-tender nodule.

A₃ c

Currently there is no link between smoking and the development of breast cancer.

A₄ e

The breast is usually dealt with through triple assessment. That is history and examination, radiological assessment (ultrasound scan or mammogram) and the histological assessment (aspiration or biopsy). In this case the patient is young and mammography would be difficult, thus an ultrasound scan is undertaken.

A₅ a

Although in 25% of cases the cause is idiopathic. In this case the patient may have developed gynaecomastia from use of spironolactone.

A₆ b

Ductal carcinoma in situ does confer an increased risk of invasive breast carcinoma – the greater the extent of the ductal carcinoma in situ, the greater the risk of invasive disease.

A₇ b

Up to 45% of breast cancers will be found in the upper outer quadrant of the breast.

A₈ d

The patient requires an urgent referral to a breast clinic for physical examination, mammography and, if appropriate, biopsy.

A₉ a

Periductal mastitis affects young women. The main complaint is mastalgia with associated nipple retraction and discharge.

A₁₀ c

This patient is suffering from periductal mastitis. It is important to treat with antibiotics to avoid progression to an abscess or a fistula.

A₁₁ d

Duct papilloma are epithelial proliferations. In younger patients they often occur in multiples and bilaterally.

A₁₂ e

While this patient is most likely suffering from an intraductal papilloma, it is difficult to distinguish from other more serious breast conditions.

A₁₃ c

While important, the liver ultrasound scan is a second-line investigation involved in the staging of breast cancer.

A₁₄ a

With just wide local excision the tumour's margins may be clear; however, this does not deal with micrometastases or any metastatic spread.

A₁₅ e

A haematoma is an early complication of radical mastectomy and is usually resolved before the patient is discharged.

A₁₆ b

Duct ectasia is the dilatation of the large breast ducts. Ageing leads to an increase in duct ectasia. It is often complicated by secondary infection.

A₁₇ c

This patient is suffering from mammary duct ectasia. For this patient the most appropriate management is analgesia and antibiotics to treat any infection. However, it can be difficult to distinguish from carcinoma and it may also warrant biopsy.

A₁₈ c

The patient's age and the fact there is a large lump with associated symptoms mean this patient is likely to be suffering from breast cancer.

A₁₉ a

This patient is most likely suffering from fat necrosis. There is often a history of trauma to the breast. However, trauma may be slight in patients with larger breasts.

A₂₀ b

While microcalcifications may indicate the natural ageing process, they can be a sign of breast carcinoma. Fine needle aspiration is the preferred investigation for breast cysts. Stereotactic biopsy allows for accurate location of the microcalcifications.

4

Vascular

Q1 A 62-year-old man has been diagnosed with severe peripheral arterial disease. You explain to the patient he should inspect his feet regularly. The following are all good places to look for evidence of early arterial insufficiency **except**?

a Heel

b Interdigital clefts

c Tips of the digits

d Dorsum of the foot

e Ulcer or wounds that do not heal

Q2 A 67-year-old has presented with a 20-minute episode of slurred speech. The patient has suffered similar episodes in the past. This patient may benefit from carotid endarterectomy. What is the next most appropriate step in management?

a Carotid angiography

b CT scan of the neck

c Doppler duplex ultrasound scan of the neck

d Magnetic resonance angiography

e Positron emission tomography

Q3 A 59-year-old woman presents to her general practitioner and is diagnosed with saphenofemoral incompetence. She had no obvious complications of her varices. Which management plan would you instigate first?

a Surgery to prevent leg ulceration

b Conservative measures

c Sclerotherapy

d Powered phlebotomy

e Endovenous obliteration

Q4 A 39-year-old female presents with a painful foot. On examination you note her foot is cold, and you cannot detect the pedal pulses. The following are all potential causes of this condition **except**?

a Arterial thrombus

b Trauma

c Atrial fibrillation

d Thrombosis secondary to plaque rupture

e Amniotic fluid embolism

Q5 The following are all correct relating to varicose veins **except**?

a More common in the short saphenous system than the long saphenous system

b Increase in incidence with age

c More common in women

d More common in those with previous deep vein thrombosis

e Patients are often disturbed by the poor cosmetic appearance

Q6 A 66-year-old man presents with gastroenteritis. During investigations he underwent a plain abdominal radiograph. It was noted he had a 4cm abdominal aortic aneurysm. After symptomatic treatment for his simple gastroenteritis he is sent home. What is the next most appropriate step in management?

a Elective surgery

b Emergency surgery

c Regular surveillance

d Start propranolol

e No management required

Q7 A 59-year-old woman requests a home visit from her general practitioner. She has a 10-year history of varicose veins. On arriving, the general practitioner immediately calls an ambulance, as she is suffering from an acute complication of her varicosities. What is the most likely diagnosis?

a Recurrent superficial thrombophlebitis

b Recent bleeding from a varicosity that has stopped

c Bleeding from a varicosity that has eroded the skin

d Progressive skin changes

e Cosmetic problems

Q8 A 74-year-old man has been diagnosed with varicose veins for 15 years. He has had little trouble with them and does not like to 'trouble the doctor'. However, he has recently developed complications of his varicosities. The following are all reasons for referral for further investigation **except**?

a Varicose eczema

b Haemosiderin discolouration

c Lipodermatosclerosis

d Venous ulceration

e Anxiety over complications

Q9 A 63-year-old man presents with severe abdominal pain. He explains that the pain started all of a sudden and is radiating to his back. He has no past medical history of note. On examination you note he looks shocked, with abdominal distension and hypotension and tachycardia. What is the most likely diagnosis?

a   A leaking abdominal aortic aneurysm

b   Renal colic

c   Acute pancreatitis

d   Acute appendicitis

e   Pyelonephritis

Q10 A 23-year-old male presents with cold, sensitive fingers and toes. He also complains of pain at rest. He has no past medical history of note but he has smoked since he was 13. What is the next most appropriate step in management?

a   Smoking cessation

b   Simple pain control

c   Amputation

d   Warfarin therapy

e   No treatment required

Q11 A 57-year-old woman has just been diagnosed with venous insufficiency of the lower limb. The consultant just quickly spoke to her and she is asking you, the house officer, for more details. The following are all recognised complications of venous insufficiency **except**?

a   Chronic ulceration

b   Deep vein thrombosis

c   Superficial phlebitis

d   Lipodermatosclerosis

e   Subcutaneous fibrosis

Q12 A 45-year-old male presents with a painful foot. He explains it is very sudden in onset and he has never experienced anything similar before. The following are all symptoms of acute limb ischaemia **except**?

a Paresthesia

b Pallor

c Palpable warmth

d Paralysis

e Pulselessness

Q13 A 57-year-old man presented with symptoms of intermittent claudication in the buttocks, pale cold legs and sexual impotence. What is the most likely diagnosis?

a Suprarenal abdominal aortic aneurysm

b Buerger's disease

c Carotid artery stenosis

d Deep vein thrombosis

e Leriche's syndrome

Q14 A 45-year-old man is rushed to hospital with a suspected leaking abdominal aortic aneurysm. The following are all potential aetiologies of his aneurysm **except**?

a Atherosclerosis

b Infection

c Takayasu's arteritis

d Ehlers–Danlos syndrome

e Trauma

Q15 A 65-year-old man presents with left leg pain. On examination you find the leg to be white, cold and pulseless. Over the next 30 minutes the leg is becoming desensate and movement in the toes is becoming difficult. It is decided to take the patient to theatre. The patient is found to have an embolus in the superficial femoral artery. Embolectomy has failed. What is the next most appropriate step in management?

a Intraoperative thrombolysis

b Pass a Fogarty balloon catheter

c Femoral-popliteal bypass

d Aorto-iliac bypass

e Above-knee amputation

Q16 A 33-year-old woman presents with sudden-onset swelling in her calf. She had recently returned from Australia. What is the next most appropriate initial investigation?

a Doppler ultrasound scan

b Duplex scanning

c VQ scan

d Venography

e Venous plethysmography

Q17 A 74-year-old male presents after a 'funny turn'. As part of his investigations he underwent a carotid Doppler study, in which he was found to have 50% narrowing at the carotid bifurcation. The following are true about carotid artery stenosis **except**?

a It may be asymptomatic

b An asymptomatic patient with narrowing of 50% or more should be offered carotid endarterectomy

c It may cause transient ischaemic attacks

d It may cause amaurosis fugax

e It may cause a thromboembolic stroke

Q18 The following are all correct relating to intermittent claudication **except?**

a It is usually caused by atherosclerosis

b It is worse at rest

c It may improve with regular exercise

d It may lead to gangrene

e Smoking cessation will improve outcome

Q19 A 56-year-old female is known to suffer from intermittent claudication and has been managed conservatively. The following are all indications to refer to a specialist service **except?**

a Development of rest pain

b Decrease in claudication distance

c Development of gangrene

d Development of arterial ulceration

e Buerger's test is negative

Q20 A 67-year-old man presents with the recent development of rest pain in both his feet. The pain worsens when he is in bed, but he can relieve the pain by dangling his feet out over the bed. What is the most likely diagnosis?

a Acute deep vein thrombosis

b Chronic venous obstruction

c Gout

d Diabetic neuropathy

e Severe peripheral vascular disease

Answers

A₁ d

The dorsum of the foot is the anterior side of the foot when in the anatomical position. While pulses may weaken over time, it is unlikely there will be obvious signs of peripheral arterial disease.

A₂ c

A Doppler ultrasound scan of the neck is a non-invasive investigation that will determine the level of stenosis of the arteries.

A₃ b

Conservative measures are usually considered first-line, especially in uncomplicated varicosities. Encourage walking and the use of elastic stockings.

A₄ e

Amniotic fluid embolism is where the amniotic fluid enters the maternal pulmonary circulation. It does not cause acute limb ischaemia.

A₅ a

Varicose veins occur with a 90% frequency in the long saphenous system, compared with 10% in the short saphenous system.

A₆ c

This patient may have been already noted to have an abdominal aortic aneurysm through the National Health Service's Abdominal Aortic Aneurysm Screening Programme. However, he should be offered regular surveillance to allow fast identification of rapidly enlarging or extending aneurysms.

A7 c

A patient with active bleeding from a site that has eroded the skin is a surgical emergency. It may not stop bleeding without surgical intervention.

A8 e

Patients should be referred to a specialist services if they develop any of the first four complications. They should hopefully undergo colour duplex ultrasound to determine the blood flow characteristics of their affected leg.

A9 a

This patient is most likely suffering from a leaking abdominal aortic aneurysm. It is a surgical emergency and this patient needs to get to theatre as soon as possible.

A10 a

This patient is suffering from thromboangiitis obliterans (Buerger's disease), a condition where there is recurrent inflammation and thrombosis of the arteries and veins of the hands and feet. It is strongly associated with smoking, and first-line therapy is for the patient to quit smoking completely. However, they may require opioid analgesia.

A11 b

While you may not regale her with all these details they are all possible complications of chronic venous insufficiency. However, deep vein thromboses are one of the causes of chronic venous insufficiency.

A12 c

An ischaemic foot will be 'perishingly' cold.

A13 e

This patient is suffering from Leriche's syndrome where there is chronic lower limb ischaemia. It is characterised by intermittent claudication in the buttocks, pale cold legs, sexual impotence and absent femoral pulses.

A₁₄ c

All of the options given are causes of aneurysms. However, Takayasu's arteritis affects the aortic arch and not the abdominal aorta. It is also most likely to affect women.

A₁₅ a

This patient should undergo intraoperative thrombolysis. If this is unsuccessful the patient may undergo a femoral-popliteal bypass. A balloon catheter should already have been tried in this situation. An aorto-iliac bypass will not help this patient. Amputation is very much a last resort.

A₁₆ a

While venography is the gold standard for detecting both above- and below-knee deep vein thromboses, the Doppler ultrasound scan is the initial investigation of choice for patients with deep vein thromboses.

A₁₇ b

Carotid artery stenosis complications can range from being asymptomatic to thromboembolic stroke. A symptomatic patient with a stenosis of 50% or more and an asymptomatic patient with stenosis of 70% or more should be offered carotid endarterectomy.

A₁₈ b

Intermittent claudication is a cramp-like, muscular pain in the calf, brought on by exercise and relieved only by rest.

A₁₉ e

Buerger's test is used to assess the adequacy of the arterial supply to the leg. If it is negative it means the arterial supply is good.

A₂₀ e

This patient is suffering from peripheral vascular disease. There is a usual progression from claudication to intermittent claudication to rest pain and then gangrene.

5

Hernias

Q1 A 43-year-old presents with acid reflux and is diagnosed with a hiatus hernia. In relation to a hiatus hernia, the following are all true **except?**

a Diagnosis can occur through endoscopy

b Severe acid reflux occurs in sliding hiatal hernias

c Sliding hiatal hernias are most common

d Treatment of choice is fundoplication

e Weight loss is advised

Q2 The following are all medial to the femoral artery **except?**

a Femoral canal

b Femoral nerve

c Femoral node

d Femoral vein

e Pubic tubercle

Q3 A 73-year-old man presents with a new lump in his groin. On examination you find an inguinal hernia. What is the most likely aetiological cause of this?

a Age

b Smoking

c Previous laparoscopic cholecystectomy

d Previous renal surgery

e Trauma

Q4 A 64-year-old man presents with a lump in his groin. On examination you note it is above and medial to the pubic tubercle. You note that on examination of the scrotum you cannot get above the mass. What is the most likely diagnosis?

a Direct inguinal hernia

b Femoral hernia

c Indirect inguinal hernia

d Lipoma

e Saphena varix

Q5 A 73-year-old woman presents with a lump in her right groin. On examination you note the lump is below and lateral to the pubic tubercle. On full examination you note there is a similar lump on the contralateral side. What is the most likely diagnosis?

a Direct inguinal hernia

b Femoral hernia

c Indirect inguinal hernia

d Lipoma

e Saphena varix

Q6 During a routine preoperative examination for a laparoscopic cholecystectomy, a 43-year-old woman is found to have a lump in her groin. The lump is below and lateral to the pubic tubercle. It is not tender or hard. What is the next most appropriate step in management?

a No treatment required

b Watch and wait

c Biopsy

d Urgent elective repair

e Urgent emergency repair

Q7 The following are all known complications of open hernia repair **except**?

a Damage to the ilioinguinal nerve

b Gas embolisation

c Recurrent hernia

d Scrotal haematoma

e Urinary retention

Q8 A 55-year-old man presents with a lump. Unfortunately he will not let you examine him fully. You manage to ascertain from his history the lump can be felt on his anterior thigh, is not painful and is not hard. The following are all common causes of groin lumps **except**?

a Inguinal hernia

b Lipoma

c Lymph node

d Saphena varix

e Obturator hernia

Q9 A 29-year-old woman presents with abdominal pain. She notes that she has felt nauseated but has not vomited. On examination the patient looks well but has a small painful mass that appears to lie in the location of the femoral canal. She is sent home. The following morning she begins to vomit and has developed a fever. The lump has now become red and acutely tender. What is the most likely diagnosis?

a Direct inguinal hernia

b Indirect inguinal hernia

c Obturator hernia

d Paraumbilical hernia

e Richter's hernia

Q10 A 27-year-old man presents with abdominal pain and vomiting. This has increased over the past 7 days. He notes there is a 1-day history of absolute constipation. Examination revealed an irreducible, tender, hot inguinal hernia with no bowel sounds. What is the most likely aetiological cause for bowel obstruction?

a Femoral hernia

b Littré's hernia

c Lumbar hernia

d Obturator hernia

e Spigelian hernia

Q11 A 75-year-old man comes to you after buying a truss to help with his direct inguinal hernia. He is confused about how to wear it properly. The following are all good recommendations **except?**

a You must not strap the truss up if part of the hernia is poking out of your tummy

b Stop wearing the truss if the hernia becomes red and tender

c Do not wear the truss at night

d You must first reduce your hernia

e You must fit it while standing up

Q12 The following are all are true in relation to a femoral hernia **except?**

a Asymptomatic femoral hernias should be treated as an urgent surgical case

b It can strangulate the bowel without obstruction

c An asymptomatic femoral hernia may contain omentum

d The femoral artery lies medial to the hernia

e It appears below and lateral to the pubic tubercle

Q13 The following are all are true in relation to an indirect inguinal hernia **except?**

   a They are more common than direct inguinal hernias

   b They are more common in women

   c They arise laterally to the inferior epigastric vessels

   d In women they follow the path of the round ligament

   e They pass through the internal inguinal ring

Q14 The following are all are true in relation to a direct inguinal hernia **except?**

   a They arise laterally to the inferior epigastric vessels

   b They push through a weakness in the posterior wall of the inguinal canal

   c They are more common in men

   d They are not covered by the internal spermatic fascia

   e They are not usually congenital

Q15 The following are all possible aetiological factors that predispose a patient to hernia formation **except?**

   a Chronic cough

   b Pregnancy

   c Regular exercise

   d Obesity

   e Persistent processus vaginalis

Q16 The following are all true about the femoral canal **except?**

   a It has the inguinal ligament as its anterior border

   b It lies lateral to the femoral vein

   c It has the pectineal ligament as it posterior border

   d It has the lacunar ligament as it medial border

   e It contains the lymph nodes of Cloquet

Q17 The following are all true about the inguinal canal **except?**

   a The roof is formed by the internal oblique and transversus abdominis

   b The floor is formed by the inguinal ligament

   c The anterior wall is formed by the aponeurosis and the superficial inguinal ring

   d The posterior wall is formed by the conjoint tendon and the deep inguinal ring

   e In males it contains the round ligament and its coverings and the ilioinguinal nerve

Q18 The following predispose a patient to an incisional hernia **except?**

   a Increased age

   b Good haemostasis

   c Malnutrition

   d Obesity

   e Wound infection

Q19 A 49-year-old male patient presents with a problem with his bowels. You enquire as to why he has surgical scars, but all he remembers was that 'two loops of my intestine got stuck in a pouch inside me'. What was his most likely diagnosis?

   a Lumbar hernia

   b Obturator hernia

   c Maydl's hernia

   d Richter's hernia

   e Spigelian hernia

Q20 An 81-year-old female presents with vomiting and colicky abdominal pain. On examination you find a small, firm and tender lump just below the inguinal ligament and lateral to the pubic tubercle. There is no cough impulse and the lump is dull to percussion. It is irreducible. What is the most likely diagnosis?

a Strangulated direct inguinal hernia

b Strangulated femoral hernia

c Strangulated indirect inguinal hernia

d Lipoma

e Saphena varix

Answers

A₁ d
Nissen fundoplication is an operation used in the treatment of intractable oesophageal reflux.

A₂ b
Remember the mnemonic NAVY, lateral to medial, nerve, artery, vein, Y-fronts.

A₃ a
The main aetiological factor of an acquired hernia is abdominal weakness caused by advancing age leading to fatty infiltration of the muscle.

A₄ c
A mass above and medial to the pubic tubercle is likely to be an inguinal hernia. If the mass then enters the scrotum it is likely to be an indirect inguinal hernia.

A₅ b
Femoral hernias are protrusion of the peritoneum into the femoral canal. They appear below and lateral to the pubic tubercle and are more common in women.

A₆ d
Femoral hernias are often asymptomatic. However, they most commonly become strangulated. Thus urgent elective repair is advised.

A₇ b
All are known complications of open hernia repair except gas embolisation, which would only occur following laparoscopic hernia repair.

A8 e

An obturator hernia is a hernia that passes through the obturator canal and which may only be felt on rectal or vaginal examination.

A9 e

This patient is suffering from a Richter's hernia. This is where the antimesenteric border (the part not attached to the mesentery) of the intestine passes through a defect in the abdominal wall (in this case the femoral canal). As only part of the intestine enters the defect, obstruction occurs relatively late.

A10 b

A Littré's hernia is the incarceration of a Meckel's diverticulum within an inguinal hernia.

A11 e

Obviously, you should fit it while the patient is lying down, as the patient needs to have the hernia reduced to fit it properly.

A12 d

The femoral artery lies lateral to the femoral canal.

A13 b

They are more common in men, as the inguinal canal is wider in males. Up to 75% of inguinal hernias are indirect.

A14 a

Direct inguinal hernias arise medially to the inferior epigastric vessels.

A15 c

Regular exercise will help keep the abdominal muscles strong.

A16 b

The femoral canal is bordered laterally by the femoral vein.

A17 e

This is true of females. In men it contains the spermatic cord, its covering and the ilioinguinal nerve.

A18 b

These are the factors that encourage good wound healing. A well-nourished, slim, young patient without a wound infection or cough will do best.

A19 c

Maydl's hernia is where two adjacent loops of small intestine are trapped within a hernia sac with a tight neck. This can lead to necrosis and ultimately requires resection to remove the damaged part. On examination the hernia is tense, tender and irreducible.

A20 b

This is a strangulated femoral hernia and requires immediate surgical intervention.

6

Urology

Q1 A 54-year-old woman is admitted with right loin pain and haematuria. On examination you note she is tender in her right loin. She undergoes a CT scan of the kidneys, ureters and bladder and this identified a right renal tract calculus. What is the most likely diagnosis?

a Renal pelvis calculus

b Mid-ureteral calculus

c Vesicoureteric calculus

d Pelvicoureteric calculus

e Bladder calculus

Q2 A 54-year-old woman is admitted with right loin pain and haematuria. On examination you note she is tender in her right loin. She undergoes a CT scan of the kidneys, ureters and bladder and this identified a right renal tract calculus. What is the most likely aetiological cause for her stone?

a Calcium oxalate

b Calcium phosphate

c Mixed oxalate/phosphate

d Struvite

e Uric acid

Q3 The following points are true in relation to urethral catheterisation **except?**

a To calculate the diameter of a Foley catheter, divide the gauge number by three

b Aseptic technique is important to avoid infection

c The male foreskin should be pulled over the glans after insertion of the catheter

d A 14F (Ch) Foley catheter is commonly used

e A povidone-iodine solution should be used as part of preparation of the urethral meatus

Q4 The following are all symptoms of the obstructive nature of benign prostatic hyperplasia **except?**

a Dribbling

b Hesitancy

c Poor stream

d Retention

e Urgency

Q5 A 66-year-old man with bony pain undergoes a radioisotope bone scan. He is found to have multiple sclerotic lesions in his axial skeleton that are thought to be metastases. What is the most likely diagnosis?

a Bladder cancer

b Breast cancer

c Lung cancer

d Prostate cancer

e Thyroid cancer

Q6 The following are all structural causes of bladder outflow obstruction **except**?

a Benign prostatic hyperplasia

b Bladder neck stenosis

c Carcinoma of the prostate

d Multiple sclerosis

e Urethral stricture

Q7 A 73-year-old man presents with symptoms of poor stream, hesitancy and nocturia. He thinks his symptoms have been getting worse over the past few months and he is fed up. After excluding more sinister causes he is diagnosed with benign prostatic hyperplasia. Which management plan would you instigate first?

a Reassurance

b Observation and review

c Commence alpha-adrenergic antagonist

d Transurethral prostatectomy

e Urethral stents

Q8 The following are all early complications following a transurethral resection of the prostate **except**?

a Epididymo-orchitis

b Extravasation

c Fluid absorption (transurethral resection syndrome)

d Incontinence

e Retrograde ejaculation

Q9 A 74-year-old man with known prostatic carcinoma presents with sudden-onset numbness and weakness in his lower limbs. He undergoes spinal surgery and is recovering well. Which management plan would you instigate first?

a Watch and wait

b Radical prostatectomy

c External beam radiotherapy alone

d Hormonal therapy alone

e Radical radiotherapy and hormonal therapy

Q10 The following are all causes of epididymo-orchitis **except**?

a Amiodarone

b Amitriptyline

c Behçet's disease

d Chlamydia trachomatis

e *Escherichia coli*

Q11 A 34-year-old man presents with a painless transilluminable swelling of his testicle. There are no other symptoms. What is the most likely diagnosis?

a Primary hydrocoele

b Testicular torsion

c Testicular tumour

d Torsion of the hydatid of Morgagni

e Varicocele

Q12 A 34-year-old man presents with a painless transilluminable swelling of his testicle. There are no other symptoms. What is the next most appropriate step in management?

a No treatment required

b Reassurance and scrotal support

c Fluid aspiration

d Exploration under anaesthetic

e Removal of testicle

Q13 A 26-year-old man presents with a painless testicular lump. On examination the lump is hard, lies within the testis and can be gotten above. It does not transilluminate. Bloods have been taken. What is the next most appropriate initial investigation?

a Chest radiograph

b CT scan of the pelvis

c Intravenous urogram

d Scrotal ultrasound scan

e Testicular biopsy

Q14 A 33-year-old man presents with a painless testicular lump. He has a past medical history of orchidopexy. He is diagnosed with a testicular tumour. What is the most likely aetiological cause for his tumour?

a Inguinal hernia

b Mumps orchitis

c Non-descent of the testis

d Physical activity

e Sedentary lifestyle

Q15 A 15-year-old boy presents with testicular pain that started after a football game 2 hours previously. On examination you find he has a tender, swollen scrotum. What is the next most appropriate step in management?

a Abdominal and testicular ultrasound scan

b Antibiotics

c Immediate surgical exploration

d No treatment required

e Watch and wait

Q16 A 15-year-old boy presents with testicular pain that started after a football game 2 hours previously. On examination you find he has a tender, swollen scrotum. Which investigation is most likely to lead to a diagnosis?

a Abdominal radiograph

b Beta-HCG

c Doppler ultrasound scan

d Radionuclide scan

e Urinalysis

Q17 The following are all indications for long-term indwelling catheterisation **except**?

a Chronic interstitial nephritis

b Neurogenic bladder

c Palliative care

d Refractory bladder outlet obstruction

e Refractory skin breakdown

Q18 The following are all contraindications for catheterisation **except?**

a Blood at the meatus

b High-riding prostate

c Trauma to the genital/perineal area (without further exploration first)

d Scrotal haematoma

e Spinal cord injury

Q19 The following are all indication for short-term indwelling catheterisation **except?**

a Acute urinary retention

b Detrusor hyperactivity

c Pelvic surgery

d Urinary output monitoring in critically ill patients

e Urological surgery

Q20 The following are all complications of long-term catheterisation **except?**

a Bacteriuria

b Calculus accretion

c Hypotension

d Pyelonephritis

e Septicaemia

Answers

A_1 c

The commonest site for calculi to sit is the vesicoureteric junction, as it is the narrowest part of the normal urinal tract.

A_2 a

Most renal tract calculi are calcium oxalate in composition.

A_3 e

Studies have shown that simple cleaning with a saline solution as part of the aseptic technique is protective against infection. Pratt RJ, Pellowe C, Loveday HP, Robinson N, *et al.* Guidelines for preventing infections associated with the insertion and maintenance of short-term indwelling urethral catheterisation in acute care. *J. Hospital Infect.* 2001; **47**: S39–S46.

A_4 e

Urgency is an irritant symptom of benign prostatic hyperplasia.

A_5 d

Osteosclerotic metastases are most commonly caused by primary prostate and breast malignancies.

A_6 d

Multiple sclerosis is a functional cause of bladder outflow obstruction.

A_7 c

In this case the patient feels he is suffering from his condition and so initial treatment is required. However, those with mild or moderate symptoms will usually be observed and reviewed.

A8 e

Retrograde is an intermediate complication following a transurethral resection of the prostate because of injury of the preprostatic sphincter system.

A9 d

This patient has metastatic disease and consequently would undergo hormonal therapy that may include strontium-89 to ease painful bony metastases.

A10 b

Amitriptyline is not a known cause of epididymo-orchitis.

A11 a

A hydrocoele is the only painless swelling that transilluminates.

A12 b

The first-line treatment for a patient with a simple primary hydrocoele is reassurance and scrotal support. However, if the patient is suffering from a secondary hydrocoele, the underlying condition must be treated.

A13 d

The patient is most likely suffering from a testicular tumour. After tumour markers the most appropriate first-line investigation is the scrotal ultrasound scan. Biopsy is not advised, as it may cause seeding of the tumour.

A14 c

This patient had suffered from cryptoorchidism. The major risk factor relating to the development of testicular cancer is an undescended testicle.

A15 c

Immediate surgical exploration is required to avoid loss of the testis.

A_{16} d

A radionuclide scan is the gold standard investigation for testicular torsion; however, it is not recommended, as if there is a high index of suspicion the patient should be taken to theatre immediately.

A_{17} a

Chronic interstitial nephritis is a complication of long-term catheterisation.

A_{18} e

Contraindications relate to urethral trauma.

A_{19} b

Detrusor hyperactivity, which occurs in those with multiple sclerosis or similar conditions, is best suited to permanent catheterisation.

A_{20} c

Hypotension is a rare complication that occurs when placing a catheter for the first time with the associated diuresis.

Orthopaedics

7

Q1 A 51-year-old man presents with an acutely swollen right knee. He states he is currently taking regular 'steroids for his asthma'. Examination reveals a hot, red and tender knee joint. He is unable to extend his knee fully. What is the most likely diagnosis?

a Bursitis

b Gout

c Pseudogout

d Ruptured Baker's cyst

e Septic arthritis

Q2 A 51-year-old man presents with an acutely swollen right knee. Examination reveals a hot, red and tender knee joint. He is unable to extend his knee fully. Which investigation is most likely to lead to a diagnosis?

a Bloods including C-reactive protein

b Bone scan

c Joint aspiration

d MRI of the knee

e Knee radiograph

Q3 A 51-year-old man presents with an acutely swollen right knee. Examination reveals a hot, red and tender knee joint. He is unable to extend his knee fully. What is the next most appropriate step in management?

a Conservative management

b Joint drainage and lavage

c Intravenous antibiotics

d Oral antibiotics

e Amputation

Q4 A 37-year-old man presents with a winged scapula. The following muscle weaknesses are not causes of a winged scapula **except**?

a Deltoid

b Levator scapula

c Pectoralis minor

d Serratus anterior

e Trapezius

Q5 A 45-year-old presents with a painful right leg. On examination you find the pain and paresthesia are localised to the medial aspect of the leg and foot (including the great toe). What is the most likely diagnosis?

a L2–L3 intervertebral disc collapse

b L3–L4 intervertebral disc collapse

c L4–L5 intervertebral disc collapse

d L5–S1 intervertebral disc collapse

e S1–S2 intervertebral disc collapse

Q6 A 35-year-old woman presents with night pain and occasional tingling in her thumb. On examination she has very slight wasting of the thenar eminence but has full power. There is equivocal sensory loss to the palmer aspect of the thumb. What is the most likely diagnosis?

a Carpal tunnel syndrome

b De Quervain's disease

c Dupuytren's contracture

d Ganglion

e Lateral epicondylitis

Q7 A 35-year-old woman presents with night pain and occasional tingling in her thumb. On examination she has very slight wasting of the thenar eminence but has full power. There is equivocal sensory loss to the palmer aspect of the thumb. What is the next most appropriate step in management?

a No treatment required

b Night splints

c Physiotherapy

d Steroid injection

e Carpal tunnel release surgery

Q8 An 83-year-old female presents to her general practitioner with sudden-onset lower back pain. It is noted she has become shorter since her last visit. Simple bloods tests reveal serum calcium, phosphorus, alkaline phosphatase and parathyroid hormone levels are all within normal limits. What is the most likely diagnosis?

a Osteitis deformans

b Osteitis fibrosis cystica

c Osteopetrosis

d Osteoporosis

e Osteomalacia

Q9 An 18-year-old woman presents 2 hours after falling on her out-stretched left hand while playing volleyball. On examination there is tenderness in the anatomical snuffbox. Wrist radiograph reveals no fracture. What is the most likely diagnosis?

a Colles' fracture

b De Quervain's disease

c Medial epicondylitis

d Scaphoid fracture

e Wrist sprain

Q10 An 18-year-old woman presents 2 hours after falling on her outstretched left hand while playing volleyball. On examination there is tenderness in the anatomical snuffbox. Wrist radiograph reveals no fracture. What is the next most appropriate step in management?

a No treatment required

b Conservative, analgesia and RICE (rest, ice, compression and elevation)

c Physiotherapy

d Upper forearm to interphalangeal joint cast

e Full arm cast

Q11 A 55-year-old man presents with an acutely swollen and painful toe. On examination you note his left great toe is swollen, erythematous and extremely tender. He is taking a number of medications to control his primary hypertension. Which investigation is most likely to lead to a diagnosis?

a Blood cultures

b Plain radiograph of his toe

c Serum uric acid

d Synovial fluid aspirate and microscopy

e Routine bloods including erythrocyte sedimentation rate

Q12 A 37-year-old woman is thrown from her horse. She has multiple injuries including a pneumothorax. A chest radiograph reveals a compound fracture of the medial clavicle. Which of the following vascular structures is particularly vulnerable in a clavicular fracture?

   a Axillary artery

   b Brachiocephalic artery

   c Lateral thoracic artery

   d Subclavian artery

   e Thoracoacromial trunk

Q13 The following are all true in regard to a Colles' fracture **except?**

   a There is dorsal angulation of the distal fragment

   b There is ventral displacement of the distal fragment

   c The is radial deviation of the hand

   d It is a transverse fracture

   e It is thought of as the dinner fork deformity

Q14 The following are all true in regard to hallux valgus **except?**

   a More common in men

   b Diagnosis can be confirmed with radiology

   c Often occurs bilaterally

   d Osteoarthritis in the first metatarsal phalangeal joint causes pain

   e Only seen in populations that wear shoes

Q15 The following are all true in regard to Achilles tendon rupture **except?**

 a It usually occurs in fit, active men

 b Sudden force to a dorsiflexed foot causes it

 c Most patients have prior Achilles tendon problems

 d In patients with an active lifestyle, surgical intervention is advised

 e There is increased risk when patients are taking fluoroquinolones

Q16 A 73-year-old woman presents with a femoral neck fracture. She is found to have a stage II fracture on the Garden's classification. What is the most likely diagnosis?

 a Incomplete fracture of the neck

 b Complete without displacement

 c Complete with partial displacement

 d Complete femoral neck fracture with full displacement

Q17 A woman presents with a femoral neck fracture. She is found to have a stage III fracture on the Garden's classification. She is a well 73-year-old and has no other co-morbidities except well-controlled hypertension. What is the next most appropriate step in management?

 a Close reduction under anaesthesia

 b Open reduction under anaesthesia

 c Dynamic hip screw

 d Austin–Moore prosthesis

 e Total hip replacement

Q18 A 93-year-old man presents after a small fall that has led to a grossly deformed leg. He also notes recent bone aches and problems with his hearing over the past year. His femur radiograph reveals a fracture through a sclerotic process. What is the most likely diagnosis?

a Bony metastases

b Hyperparathyroidism

c Osteomyelitis

d Paget's disease

e Primary bone tumour

Q19 The following are all possible complications of a scaphoid fracture **except**?

a Avascular necrosis

b Malunion

c Non-union

d Osteoarthritis

e Osteoporosis

Q20 A 75-year-old man presents with wasting of the intrinsic muscles of the hand. The following are all possible causes **except**?

a Brachial plexus injury

b Carpal tunnel syndrome

c Motor neurone disease

d Pancoast's tumour

e Syringomyelia

Answers

A₁ e

A hot, acutely swollen, tender joint is assumed to be septic arthritis until proven otherwise. Untreated septic arthritis can destroy a joint within days. In adults it is associated with immunosuppression and the knee joint.

A₂ c

The definitive investigation is joint aspiration. It is important to undertake the aspiration before commencing treatment.

A₃ c

Intravenous antibiotics should be started empirically and adjusted if required after antibiotic sensitivity has been determined. Antibiotic therapy should continue for 6 weeks.

A₄ d

This is often caused by lesions of the long thoracic nerve. The serratus anterior holds the scapula against the thoracic wall.

A₅ b

The dermatome affected is in the distribution of L4.

A₆ a

Carpal tunnel syndrome is the entrapment of the median nerve, which causes the symptoms and signs listed here.

A₇ b

As she is suffering from mostly pain at night, night splints may be most helpful. If this does not work, then further treatment could be sought.

A8 d

Osteoporosis is the most likely culprit. She has lost height, she has associated back pain (most likely crush fractures) and her blood results are normal.

A9 d

While there is no fracture visible on the radiograph, scaphoid fractures are usually only visible after 7–10 days. Pain in the anatomical snuffbox is highly indicative of a scaphoid fracture.

A10 d

This patient is suspected to have a scaphoid fracture. Thus, the wrist is immobilised and should be reassessed at 10 days.

A11 d

While the urate level may be raised, it is more likely to be normal during an acute flare. Therefore, synovial fluid aspiration would show negatively birefringent crystals if the patient was suffering from gout.

A12 d

The subclavian is most vulnerable in this position. The maxillary artery is more vulnerable in anterior dislocations of the humerus.

A13 b

There is dorsal displacement of the distal fragment.

A14 a

It is more common in women.

A15 c

Most patients (up to 80%) do not suffer from prior Achilles problems.

A16 b

Garden's classification does not relate to femoral neck fractures.

A17 d

Remember the mnemonic for Garden fractures 1,2 plate and screw; 3,4 Austin–Moore.

A18 d

Slight trauma causes fracture in Paget's bone because of the disorganised bone architecture.

A19 e

Osteoporosis is not caused by fractures.

A20 b

Wasting of the small muscles of the hand is due to a lesion affecting the ulnar nerve. Carpal tunnel syndrome is due to entrapment of the median nerve. The median nerve supplies the LOAF muscles (**L**ateral two lumbricals, **O**pponens pollicis, **A**bductor pollicis brevis and **F**lexor pollicis brevis).

8

Ear, nose and throat

Q1 The following are symptoms and signs of an acoustic neuroma **except?**

a Facial droop

b Loss of the corneal reflex

c Occipital pain on the side of the tumour

d Tinnitus

e Unilateral sensorineural deafness

Q2 A 19-year-old woman presents with a sore throat. She has been suffering from dysphagia and has been feeling generally unwell. On examination you note she is pyrexial, with enlarged tonsils that are exuding pus. Her pharyngeal mucosa is inflamed and her cervical lymph nodes are large and tender. Her bloods show an increased neutrophil count. She is also Paul–Bunnell negative. What is the diagnosis?

a Acute tonsillitis

b Diphtheria

c Infectious mononucleosis

d Mumps

e Quinsy

Q3 The following are all indications for tonsillectomy **except?**

    a Acute tonsillitis

    b Chronic tonsillitis

    c Quinsy

    d Sleep apnoea

    e Tonsillar malignancy

Q4 The following are all types of acquired paediatric stridor **except?**

    a Epiglottitis

    b Impacted foreign body

    c Laryngomalacia

    d Laryngotracheobronchitis

    e Vocal cord palsy

Q5 A 4-year-old presents to the emergency department. She looks very unwell and is unable to talk. Her cough sounds like a quack. You note she is drooling and has stridor. What is the most likely diagnosis?

    a Acute asthma

    b Acute tonsillitis

    c Croup

    d Epiglottitis

    e Impacted foreign body

Q6 A 4-year-old presents to the emergency department. She looks unwell and is unable to talk. Her cough sounds like a quack. You note she is drooling and has stridor. Which management plan would you instigate first?

a Examine the throat and fast-bleep the ear, nose and throat surgeon and the anaesthetics registrar

b Start antibiotics and nebulisers and fast-bleep the ear, nose and throat surgeon and the anaesthetics registrar

c Start nebulised adrenaline and fast-bleep the ear, nose and throat surgeon and the anaesthetics registrar

d Commence rapid sequence induction

e Emergency tracheostomy

Q7 A 23-year-old man was playing a drinking game with his friends. This led to him 'ingesting' a 2 pence piece into his aerodigestive tract. He is breathing well. His posteroanterior chest radiograph shows the offending coin as an opaque circle in line with the first few thoracic vertebrae. What is the most likely diagnosis?

a Coin is in the oesophagus at the level of the cricopharyngeus

b Coin is in the oesophagus at the level of the aortic arch

c Coin is in the oesophagus at the level of the lower oesophageal sphincter

d Coin is in the right main bronchus

e Coin is in the stomach

Q8 What is the most likely aetiological cause for an acute painful swelling of the parotid gland in children?

a Calculus

b Cyst

c Infectious mononucleosis

d Mumps

e Sjögren's syndrome

Q9 A 37-year-old man presents with a painless swelling on the side of his face. On examination you note a mass, 4 × 3 × 2 cm, overlying the angle of the mandible and which is not fixed to over- or under-lying structures. Cranial nerve examination is normal. What is the most likely diagnosis?

a Acinic cell carcinoma

b Adenocarcinoma

c Lipoma

d Pleomorphic adenoma

e Squamous cell carcinoma

Q10 A 33-year-old woman presents with an asymmetrical face. On examination you find she has a unilateral drooping of the right side of her face. However, she is still able to wrinkle her forehead and raise her eyebrows. What is the most likely diagnosis?

a Cranial nerve V palsy

b Cranial nerve VII upper motor neurone palsy

c Cranial nerve VII lower motor neurone palsy

d Cranial nerve VIII palsy

e Cranial nerve IX palsy

Answers

A₁ a

Involvement of the seventh cranial nerve occurs after surgery.

A₂ a

The classic presentation of acute tonsillitis.

A₃ a

While recurrent tonsillitis is a relative indication for tonsillectomy, one episode is not.

A₄ c

Laryngomalacia is congenital.

A₅ d

This child is suffering from epiglottitis.

A₆ c

Do not examine the throat. It is likely to become obstructed. This is an ear, nose and throat emergency. The nebulised adrenaline may allow the ear, nose and throat surgeon and anaesthetics registrar time to arrive and treat the child. Rapid sequence induction involves paralysis, and if intubation is difficult it would abolish the airway.

A₇ b

Remember when looking at the radiograph, coins which have become lodged in the oesophagus will usually appear as a radiopaque circle whereas the tracheal rings lead to the coin being trapped horizontally. O = Oesophagus; — = Trachea.

A8 d

Common in children (despite vaccination with mumps, measles and rubella vaccine because of lack of herd immunity). It may be unilateral or it may affect the submandibular glands.

A9 d

Pleomorphic adenomas are the most common type of parotid tumour. Normal cranial nerve examination implies no local invasion or malignancy.

A10 b

There is bilateral control of the upper facial muscles (frontalis and orbicularis oculi).

9

Neck

Q₁ A 19-year-old woman presents with an enlarging lump in her neck. On examination it lies in the upper third of the anterior triangle. It is fluctuant in nature. What is the most likely diagnosis?

a Branchial cyst

b Carotid body tumour

c Cystic hygroma

d Lymph node

e Thyroid cyst

Q₂ A 24-year-old man presents with a new swelling in his neck. On examination you find a mass 2 × 2 cm in size in the anterior triangle of the neck. It is not fixed to underlying structures and it is tender. You find no other signs. What is the most likely diagnosis?

a Branchial cyst

b Carotid artery aneurysm

c Dermoid cyst

d Lymph node

e Thyroglossal cysts

Q3 A 24-year-old man presents with a new swelling in his neck. On examination you find a mass in the posterior triangle of the neck. It is soft and non-tender. You can palpate the mass anteriorly away from the neck. On examination of his hands you note slight wasting of the thenar eminence. Which investigation is most likely to lead to a diagnosis?

a Angiography

b Chest radiograph

c CT scan of the brain

d Electromyography

e Full blood count

Q4 A 78-year-old man presents with a nosebleed that has continued for 2 hours. He had a similar episode yesterday that stopped spontaneously. What is the next most appropriate step in management?

a No treatment required

b Apply pressure

c Apply 1:1000 adrenaline to Little's area

d Cauterise with silver nitrate stick

e Nasal tampon packing

Q5 A 78-year-old man presents with a nosebleed that has continued for 2 hours. He had a similar episode yesterday that stopped spontaneously. What is the next most appropriate initial investigation?

a No further investigation required

b Monitor vital signs 4-hourly

c Blood count, clotting screen and crossmatch

d Radiograph facial bones

e CT scan of the head

Q6 The following are all immediate complications of thyroidectomy **except?**

a Haemorrhage

b Hypocalcaemia

c Laryngeal oedema

d Recurrent laryngeal nerve damage

e Thyroid storm

Q7 A 23-year-old British woman is diagnosed with thyroid cancer. Of note, she has also been suffering from diarrhoea and facial flushing. Her mother has also suffered from the same cancer. What is the most likely diagnosis?

a Anaplastic carcinoma

b Follicular carcinoma

c Medullary carcinoma

d Papillary carcinoma

e Thyroid lymphoma

Q8 A 27-year-old woman presents with a mass in her neck. Which investigation is most likely to lead to a diagnosis?

a Chest radiograph

b Fine needle biopsy

c Thyroid scanning with radioiodine

d Serum thyroglobulin

e Ultrasound scan of the neck

Q9 A 27-year-old woman presents with 'asthma'. She explains she has had problems breathing and that this worsens when she is doing yoga and her arms are raised above her head. You ask her to raise her arms above her head and this leads to facial congestion and stridor. The following are all causes of this specific sign **except**?

a Aortic aneurysm

b Cervical rib

c Globus pharyngeus

d Lymphoma

e Retrosternal goitre

Q10 A 27-year-old woman presents with 'asthma'. She explains she has had problems breathing and that this worsens when she is doing yoga and her arms are raised above her head. You ask her to raise her arms above her head and this leads to facial congestion and stridor. Which investigation is most likely to lead to a diagnosis?

a Fine needle biopsy of the neck

b Plain radiograph of the neck and thoracic inlet

c Radioiodine scan

d Thyroid function tests

e Ultrasound scan of the neck

Answers

A1 a
A branchial cyst lies in the anterior triangle. It is a remnant of the branchial complex and classically presents before the patient is 30 years old.

A2 d
A lymph node is the most likely cause of swelling in the neck.

A3 b
A chest radiograph will reveal the cervical rib causing thoracic outlet syndrome.

A4 b
The first-line therapy is to apply pressure.

A5 c
After initial clinical assessment it is important to assess blood count and clotting factors.

A6 b
Remember: primary complications occur during the operation, reactionary or early are within 24 hours, and late occur after 24 hours.

A7 c
In 20% of cases, medullary carcinoma is autosomally inherited.

A8 b
The most effective method of distinguishing benign from malignant nodules.

A9 c

This is known as Pemberton's sign and is a test for thoracic inlet obstruction.

A10 b

The plain radiograph will show a radiopaque mass in the retrosternal location.

10

Trauma

Q1 A 45-year-old man presents following a road traffic collision with another car at 30 mph. He was not wearing his seatbelt and he has extensive facial injuries. He also appears to have blood coming out from his right ear. He is not talking and appears to have difficulty in breathing. What is the next most appropriate step in management?

a Chin lift, jaw thrust and hard collar

b Nasopharyngeal airway

c Guedel airway (oropharyngeal airway)

d Endotracheal intubation

e Cricothyroidotomy

Q2 A 45-year-old man presents following a road traffic collision with another car at 30 mph. He was not wearing his seatbelt. The following are all injuries that should be identified during the primary survey **except**?

a Aortic disruption

b Airway obstruction

c Flail chest

d Open pneumothorax

e Tension pneumothorax

Q3 An 18-year-old man presents after being stabbed several times in the abdomen. Most of his wounds were fairly superficial. During his recovery it becomes apparent that he has developed a direct inguinal hernia. What is the most likely diagnosis?

a Genitofemoral nerve damage

b Ilioinguinal nerve damage

c Iliohypogastric nerve (lateral cutaneous branch) damage

d Lateral cutaneous nerve damage

e Obturator nerve damage

Q4 A 45-year-old woman presents with a headache. On further questioning she describes it as 'the worst headache she has ever had'. She denies any trauma. On examination she is hypertensive, photophobic and has neck stiffness. Fundal examination is difficult. What is the most likely diagnosis?

a Extradural haemorrhage

b Meningitis

c Migraine

d Subarachnoid haemorrhage

e Subdural haemorrhage

Q5 A 45-year-old woman presents with a sudden-onset headache that started 4 hours previously. On further questioning she describes it as 'the worst headache she has ever had'. She denies any trauma. On examination she is photophobic and has neck stiffness. Fundal examination is difficult and inconclusive. What is the next most appropriate initial investigation?

a CT scan of the brain

b Cerebral angiography

c MRI of the brain

d Lumbar puncture

e Routine bloods

Q6 A 23-year-old man is playing cricket when he is struck on the side of his head by the ball. He falls to the ground but does not lose consciousness. He wants to continue because he is close to 50 runs. While at afternoon tea he develops a slight headache and takes simple analgesia. At the close of play he develops a severe headache, he begins to vomit and he is obviously confused. What is his most likely diagnosis?

a Bleeding from torn bridging veins

b Contrecoup injury

c Rupture of a pre-existing berry aneurysm

d Rupture of an arteriovenous malformation

e Transection of a branch of the middle meningeal artery

Q7 A 23-year-old man is playing cricket when he is struck on the side of his head by the ball. He falls to the ground but does not lose consciousness. He wants to continue because he is close to 50 runs. While at afternoon tea he develops a slight headache and takes simple analgesia. As the game ends for the day he develops a severe headache, he begins to vomit and he is obviously confused. As he is being examined, his consciousness level drops to 9 on the Glasgow Coma Scale. What is the next most appropriate step in management?

a Craniotomy

b CT scan

c Emergency burr hole

d Lumbar puncture

e MRI

Q_8 A 45-year-old woman has reached 24 hours after the operation for her total thyroidectomy. She suddenly becomes breathless. You are called to see her and she has an obvious stridor and her oxygen saturations are dropping. Her lungs are clear. What is the next most appropriate step in management?

a   Arterial blood gas

b   Chest radiograph

c   Furosemide (40 mg)

d   Rapid sequence induction

e   Remove her sutures

Q_9 You are flying back to the UK from Australia when the captain asks if there is a doctor on board the plane. You find a tall 24-year-old man with breathing difficulties. He explains slowly that he has chest pain and breathing difficulties that came on suddenly. You try to examine as best you can. He is dyspnoeic, you think he has reduced breath sounds on the right side and his trachea appears to deviate to the left. What is the diagnosis?

a   Asthma

b   Panic attack

c   Pulmonary embolism

d   Simple pneumothorax

e   Tension pneumothorax

Q10 You are flying back to the UK from Australia when the captain asks if there is a doctor on board the plane. You find a tall 24-year-old man with breathing difficulties. He explains slowly that he has chest pain and breathing difficulties that came on suddenly. You try to examine as best you can. He is dyspnoeic, you think he has reduced breath sounds on the right side and his trachea appears to deviate to the left. What is the next most appropriate step in management?

a Administer oxygen and review

b Attach an automatic external defibrillator device

c Insert a wide-bore needle attached to the largest syringe available (half-filled with sterile liquid) into the second intercostal space in the midclavicular line

d Insert a wide-bore needle attached to the largest syringe available (half-filled with sterile liquid) into the fifth intercostal space in the midaxillary line

e Perform cricothyroidotomy

Q11 A 45-year-old man presents with severe epigastric pain for the past 6 hours. On examination the patient is very still and looks unwell. His pulse is 113 beats per minute, his blood pressure is 135/90 and he is breathing shallowly. His abdomen is tender and rigid with guarding. Bowel sounds are present. What is the most likely diagnosis?

a Acute cholecystitis

b Acute gastroenteritis

c Acute pancreatitis

d Perforated colonic diverticulum

e Perforated peptic ulcer

Q12 A 45-year-old man presents with severe epigastric pain for the past
6 hours. On examination the patient is very still and looks unwell.
His pulse is 113 beats per minute, his blood pressure is 135/90
and he is breathing shallowly. His abdomen is tender and rigid
with guarding. Bowel sounds are present. He is started on fluid
resuscitation and routine bloods are taken. What is the next most
appropriate step in management?

a CT scan of the abdomen

b Erect chest radiograph

c Electrocardiograph

d Gastroscopy

e Wait and watch, with simple analgesia

Q13 You are called to see a 31-year-old male recovering from an open
reduction and internal fixation of a compound tibial fracture (it
is 24 hours after the operation), as he has suddenly developed
increasing pain in his leg despite regular analgesia. On examination, the toes are pale (the rest of the leg is covered in surgical
dressings). It is exquisitely painful on passive movement and muscle palpation. However, you have difficulty detecting peripheral
pulses. What is the next most appropriate step in management?

a Increase analgesia

b Increase analgesia and monitor

c Remove all dressings and other constrictive items and
monitor

d Open fasciotomy

e Amputation

Q14 A 15-year-old boy presents 12 hours after an accident in a field on his father's dairy farm. What started as a minor abrasion has now become much worse. The skin around the abrasion is beginning to darken and is starting to slough off with a foul-smelling exudate. There is palpable crepitus over the thigh. What is the most likely aetiological cause for this development?

a *Actinomyces israelii*

b *Clostridium welchii*

c *Clostridium tetani*

d *Staphylococcus aureus*

e *Streptococcus pyogenes*

Q15 A 35-year-old woman presents after following a suicide attempt and has deep lacerations to her wrist. The following are all possible sequelae **except**?

a Loss of sensation to the nail beds of the radial three and a half fingers

b Loss of thumb abduction

c Loss of thumb flexion

d Loss of the extension of the first interphalangeal joint

e Wrist drop

Q16 A 73-year-old man is brought to the emergency department unconscious. His wife details a month's history of headaches, confusion and memory loss. She denies serious trauma but recalls he hit his head when playing with the grandchildren. What is the most likely diagnosis?

a Extradural haematoma

b Cerebrovascular accident

c Subarachnoid haemorrhage

d Subdural haematoma

e Vertebral dissection

Q17 A 67-year-old man presents with sudden-onset severe epigastric pain that radiates to the back. On examination his blood pressure is 88/60 and his pulse rate is 113. The following are all possible courses of action **except**?

a CT scan of the abdomen

b Gain intravenous access with two large-bore catheters

c Maintenance of blood pressure to 120/80

d Advise theatre for emergency laparotomy

e Ultrasound scan of the abdomen

Q18 A 34-year-old man presents with a penetrating chest injury. During the primary survey you note the patient has blood pressure of 90/60, his heart sounds are muffled and his jugular veins are distended. What is the most likely diagnosis?

a Cardiac contusion

b Cardiac tamponade

c Pulmonary contusion

d Tension pneumothorax

e Traumatic aortic disruption

Q19 A 34-year-old man presents with a penetrating chest injury. During the primary survey you note the patient has blood pressure of 90/60, his heart sounds are muffled and his jugular veins are distended. What is the next most appropriate step in management?

a Routine bloods and observation

b Cardioversion at 360J

c Chest drain insertion

d CT scan of the thorax

e Pericardiocentesis

Q20 A 23-year-old woman presents following her horse kicking her chest. On examination of her chest, you note on inspiration a segment of her chest is drawn inwards. What is the most likely diagnosis?

a Cardiac contusion

b Cardiac tamponade

c Flail chest

d Simple pneumothorax

e Tension pneumothorax

Q21 A 23-year-old woman presents following her horse kicking her chest. On examination of her chest, you note on inspiration a segment of her chest is drawn inwards. The following are all possible complications of such an injury **except**?

a Increased tidal volume

b Haemothorax

c Pneumothorax

d Pulmonary contusion

e Respiratory failure

Q22 A 19-year-old man presents with a sudden onset of pain in his left testis. He has vomited three times in the past hour. On examination the testis is red and swollen. Gentle lifting of the affected testicle does not relieve the pain. What is the most likely diagnosis?

a Epididymo-orchitis

b Strangulated inguinal hernia

c Testicular torsion

d Testicular tumour

e Torsion of the hydatid of Morgagni

Q23 A 65-year-old man presents with haematemesis. This is his third presentation of this kind in the past 2 years. His past two admissions were because of oesophageal variceal bleeding. The following are all used to calculate his mortality risk from this episode of bleeding **except?**

a Age

b Liver cirrhosis

c Diagnosis

d Previous haematemesis

e Pulse

Q24 The following are all indications for immediate thoracotomy within the confines of the emergency department **except?**

a Abdominal haemorrhage requiring aortic cross-clamping

b Acute pericardial tamponade in the unstable patient

c Internal cardiac massage

d Large (>1500 mL) output from chest drainage

e Rapidly exsanguinating intrathoracic haemorrhage

Q25 A 52-year-old female is hypotensive, with a blood pressure of 80/60, 12 hours after an operation. You think this patient requires a fluid challenge. What is the next most appropriate step in management?

a 1 L of 5% dextrose over 4 hours

b 1 L of normal saline over 4 hours

c 1 unit of packed red cells over 1 hour

d 250 mL of Gelofusine over 1 hour

e 500 mL of normal saline over 10 minutes

Answers

A₁ e
In this case a cricothyroidotomy is the only choice. Extensive facial injury with basal skull fracture rules out the other choices.

A₂ a
While there may be circulatory issues in such a patient, this would not be identified at the primary survey.

A₃ b
The ilioinguinal nerve innervates the portion of the internal oblique muscle that inserts into the lateral border of the conjoint tendon.

A₄ d
'The worst headache of my life' and meningism = subarachnoid haemorrhage until proven otherwise.

A₅ a
A CT scan is the investigation of choice.

A₆ e
This patient had a blow to the side of his head and this is in keeping with the most common cause of extradural haemorrhage, which is transection of a branch of the middle meningeal artery.

A₇ c
This patient required an emergency burr hole to provide temporary relief before proceeding to craniotomy to evacuate the haematoma.

A₈ e

This is a surgical emergency. She is suffering from a haematoma that is compressing the airway. You must remove her sutures immediately.

A₉ e

This patient has a tension pneumothorax. The trachea is deviated away from the side of the pain and the collapsed lung and he is breathless.

A₁₀ c

This patient is suffering from a tension pneumothorax. Most commercial long-haul airlines will carry needles and syringes. However, this is only a short-term solution and so the plane needs to lower its altitude and land as quickly as possible.

A₁₁ e

The most likely diagnosis is a perforated peptic ulcer. Epigastric pain with rigidity and guarding indicates a perforated viscus. His age makes the peptic ulcer more likely.

A₁₂ b

An erect chest radiograph would be the best choice to show air under the diaphragm. Gastroscopy is contraindicated to avoid further damage and more stomach contents will enter the peritoneal cavity.

A₁₃ c

The first thing that should be done in this patient is the removal of all constrictive dressings. The limb should be closely monitored and compartment pressure should be measured. If the pressure increases then proceed to fasciotomy.

A₁₄ b

The most common cause of gas gangrene is *Clostridium perfringens* (formerly known as *C. welchii*), which is found in soil and animal faeces.

A₁₅ e

Wrist drop is as a result of a radial nerve lesion.

A₁₆ d
The most likely diagnosis is a chronic subdural haematoma, a history of minor trauma leading to rupture of the cortical bridging veins, which causes a slow bleed.

A₁₇ c
While it is important to ensure adequate fluid volume, the patient should be maintained with a systolic of less than 100 mmHg to ensure no further rupture or dislodgement of any thrombus formed.

A₁₈ b
This is the classic presentation of cardiac tamponade known as Beck's triad.

A₁₉ e
Cardiac tamponade is an emergency. The pericardium should be drained as soon as possible. This is usually accomplished through pericardiocentesis unless other facilities for direct visualisation are available. If the patient is unstable, thoracotomy may be undertaken.

A₂₀ c
This patient is suffering from a flail segment – these cause paradoxical respiration.

A₂₁ a
There will be a decrease in tidal volume.

A₂₂ c
This is a surgical emergency. While ultrasound may reveal reduced arterial flow, the patient should be sent for surgical exploration as soon as possible.

A₂₃ d
The Rockall score deals with age, signs of shock, co-morbidities, diagnosis on endoscopy and stigmata of recent haemorrhage.

A₂₄ d

The emergency department undertakes procedures for immediately life-threatening injuries. While 1500 mL is a large output from chest drainage, it is not immediately life-threatening, but it can be carried out urgently.

A₂₅ e

Depending upon local guidelines, a fluid challenge consists of 250 mL of colloid or 500 mL of crystalloid. It should be administered quickly and a response should be seen within minutes.

Extended matching questions

Questions 1–20

Q₁

a Benign colonic structure

b Colorectal cancer

c Diverticular disease

d Haemorrhoids

e Hyperthyroidism

f Infectious diarrhoea

g Inflammatory bowel disease

h Irritable bowel syndrome

i Ischaemic colitis

j Radiation proctitis

For each of the patients below, choose the **single** most likely cause of the symptoms from the above list of options. Each option may be used once, more than once or not at all.

1 A 27-year-old woman presents complaining of bloating and excessive flatus. She is passing pellet-like stools associated with abdominal pains. Her symptoms have been intermittent for several years.

2 A 73-year-old man presents with a 5-month history of straining with bowel movements. He also feels that he cannot empty his rectum completely. He is passing blood and mucus per rectum. He has some weight loss and anorexia.

3 A 19-year-old man presents with a 4-week history of passing bloody liquid stools with mucus 10 times a day. He has anorexia, weight loss and anaemia.

4 A 19-year-old man presents having returned from a recent backpacking holiday in India. He passes bloody liquid stools about 10 times a day. He is pyrexial, anorexic and nauseated.

5 A 65-year-old man had an elective aortic aneurysm repair 5 days ago. He now has abdominal distension and left-sided abdominal pain. He is passing a small amount of blood and mucus per rectum.

Q₂

a	Glandular fever	e	Mumps
b	Hodgkin's lymphoma	f	Parotitis
c	Lymphadenopathy secondary to infection	g	Pharyngeal pouch
		h	Thyroglossal cyst
d	Lymphadenopathy secondary to malignancy	i	Thyroid cancer
		j	Thyroiditis

For each of the patients below, choose the **single** most likely cause of the symptoms from the above list of options. Each option may be used once, more than once or not at all.

1 An 80-year-old man presents with dysphagia. He has a 60 pack-year history of smoking. On examination there is a reducible mass over the lateral aspect of his neck.

2 An anxious 47-year-old woman presents with a lump in the neck. She has lost 3 kg in 3 months. On examination there is nodular enlargement of the thyroid gland on both sides of the neck.

3 A 53-year-old man presents with a painful lump in his neck. He explains he had a 'cold' last week. On examination you note a hard mobile lump in the supraclavicular fossa.

4 A 19-year-old man presents with a 7-day history of fever, tiredness and pain on swallowing. He is worried because he has found lumps in his neck. On examination you also note a tender scrotal swelling.

5 A 15-year-old girl presents with a midline swelling of the neck that has recently become tender. On examination the lump moves on swallowing and with protrusion of the tongue.

Q₃

a	Acute pancreatitis	f	Mallory–Weiss tear
b	Divarication of the recti	g	Oesophageal varices
c	Fractured rib	h	Pancreatic pseudocyst
d	Haematoma of the rectus sheath	i	Splenic rupture
e	Hepatoma	j	Umbilical hernia

For each of the patients below, choose the **single** most likely cause of the symptoms from the above list of options. Each option may be used once, more than once or not at all.

1　A 50-year-old man who is alcohol dependent presents with nausea, vomiting and epigastric pain. He has avoided attending the hospital on a number of occasions. On examination he has a palpable epigastric mass and a raised amylase. A CT scan shows a round, well-circumscribed mass in the epigastrium.

2　A 40-year-old multiparous woman presents with a midline abdominal mass. The mass in non-tender and appears when she is straining. On examination, you note there is a non-tender midline mass that is visible when she raises her head off the examining bed.

3　A 19-year-old man presents with sudden severe upper abdominal pain after being tackled during rugby practice. Past medical history includes a recent diagnosis of glandular fever.

4　A 7-year-old girl presents with spontaneous massive haematemesis. On examination you note splenomegaly.

5　A 55-year-old man with a history of alcohol dependency presents with vomiting 500 mL of blood. His blood pressure is 80/50 and his pulse rate is 120. On examination you note the patient has ascites.

Q4

a Anterior shoulder dislocation

b Calcaneal fracture

c Colles' fracture

d Galeazzi fracture

e Greenstick fracture

f March fracture

g Posterior shoulder dislocation

h Scaphoid fracture

i Spiral fracture of the tibia

j Supracondylar fracture of the humerus

For each of the patients below, choose the **single** most likely cause of the symptoms from the above list of options. Each option may be used once, more than once or not at all.

1 A 33-year-old man with a history of epilepsy presents by ambulance following a fit and is now unable to move his right arm and shoulder. On preliminary examination you note he is supporting the arm in internal rotation with the other hand.

2 A 26-year-old woman sustains a twisting injury to her left leg while skiing. She has mid-calf swelling and tenderness and is unable to bear weight on the affected leg.

3 A 7-year-old girl falls and sustains an injury to her right arm. The forearm is stiff, and the hand is deformed. She is only able to extend her fingers when her wrist is passively flexed.

4 A 33-year-old man who is a long-distance runner complains of pain in the second toe. He ran his last marathon a week ago.

5 A 21-year-old woman falls onto her outstretched hands. She complains of pain and decreased mobility of her right wrist. On examination she is tender in the anatomical snuffbox.

Q5

a Closed thoracostomy tube drainage

b Debridement and repair

c Endotracheal intubation

d Nasogastric tube suction and observation

e Observation and angiography

f Peritoneal lavage

g Pressure dressing

h Surgical repair of the extensor digitorum muscle

i Surgical repair of the flexor digitorum profundus tendon

j Urgent surgical exploration

For each of the patients below, choose the **single** most appropriate management from the above list of options. Each option may be used once, more than once or not at all.

1 A 19-year-old man presents to the emergency department by ambulance after being stabbed in the neck. He complains of difficulty swallowing and talking. He has no stridor. On examination, there is a small penetrating wound with diffuse neck swelling.

2 An 11-year-old boy presents with a hand injury sustained while playing rugby and attempting to catch the ball. On examination he is unable to bend the tip of his right middle finger.

3 A 37-year-old woman is brought into the emergency department by ambulance following a road traffic incident. On examination she has a respiratory rate of 50 breaths per minute. She has no breath sounds on the left side of her chest and her trachea is deviated to the right.

4 A 23-year-old man sustains a stab wound to the right thigh. On examination, he has a large haematoma over the thigh and weak distal pulses. He is unable to move his foot and complains of pins and needles in his foot.

5 A 45-year-old woman is involved in a road traffic accident as a passenger wearing a seatbelt. She presents with diffuse abdominal pain. She undergoes an upright chest X-ray, which shows elevation of the diaphragm with what appears to be a stomach gas bubble in the left lower lung field.

Q₆

a Benign polyps

b Crohn's disease

c Duodenal ulcer

d Gastric ulcer

e Mallory–Weiss tear

f Meckel's diverticulitis

g Oesophageal malignancy

h Oesophageal varices

i Oesophagitis

j Ulcerative colitis

For each of the patients below, choose the **single** most likely cause of the symptoms from the above list of options. Each option may be used once, more than once or not at all.

1 A 43-year-old woman who has been taking ibuprofen as pain relief for migraines presents to the emergency department complaining of black tarry stools and pain in her stomach. On further questioning she also notes the pain is worse on eating.

2 A 25-year-old Jewish man presents to the emergency department with some abdominal discomfort, weight loss with associated loss of appetite, a history of diarrhoea and bloody stools.

3 A 36-year-old man presents with a 36-hour history of diarrhoea and vomiting following a takeaway meal the day before. In the last few hours he has increasing amounts of bright red blood in his vomit.

4 An 80-year-old man presents with a 6-month history of increasing weakness and a 10 kg weight loss, vague abdominal pain and some episodes of black stools. He appears cachectic. He is a long-term smoker.

5 A 2-year-old boy is brought in by his parents with a history of painless red blood being passed per rectum. Blood tests reveal an iron-deficiency anaemia.

Q7

a	Barium enema	f	*Helicobacter pylori* antibodies
b	Barium meal	g	History only
c	Colonoscopy	h	Serum amylase
d	Full blood count, erythrocyte sedimentation rate, creatinine, electrolytes and liver function tests	i	Stool examination for pathogens
		j	Ultrasound scan of the abdomen
e	Gastroscopy		

For each of the patients below, choose the **single** most appropriate investigation from the above list of options. Each option may be used once, more than once or not at all.

1   A 70-year-old man with an 80 pack-year history of smoking complains of a 7-week history of epigastric discomfort that is worse on eating. He has lost his appetite, as he has a sense of fullness all the time, and he has lost 5 kg. You find his abdominal examination unremarkable.

2   A 45-year-old man presents with increasingly severe central abdominal pain over the last 3 hours. The pain radiates through his back and has made him vomit. He has no previous medical history. On examination he is cold and sweaty, his pulse is 130 and his blood pressure is 85/70. You also note guarding over his whole abdomen.

3   A 20-year-old woman complains of abdominal discomfort and bloating over the last 3 months. She also has intermittent diarrhoea, but her symptoms are relieved when she opens her bowels. There is no blood or mucus in her stools. Abdominal and rectal examination is normal.

4   A 50-year-old woman has sudden severe epigastric pain that radiates to the back on the right and she has been vomiting. Examination is difficult, as her body mass index score is 37, but you think she has some guarding over the epigastrium and right hypochondrium.

5   A 25-year-old previously well man has a 3-day history of abdominal cramps and diarrhoea with bloody stools five or six times a day. Examination shows a soft but tender abdomen.

Q8

a Acute pancreatitis	g Perforated peptic ulcer
b Aortic dissection	h Ruptured aortic aneurysm
c Appendicitis	
d Diverticulitis	i Small bowel obstruction
e Meckel's diverticulum	j Ulcerative colitis
f Mesenteric infarction	

For each of the patients below, choose the **single** most likely cause of the symptoms from the above list of options. Each option may be used once, more than once or not at all.

1   A 70-year-old man presents with a 2-day history of constipation, anorexia and pain in his side. On examination, he is pyrexial and there is localised tenderness and rebound in the left iliac fossa. His white blood cell count is 14.0×10^9/L.

2   A 50-year-old man presents with a 24-hour history of sudden onset of severe epigastric pain, which has now become generalised. On examination he has pyrexia, a rigid abdomen and absent bowel sounds. His white blood cell count is 18.0×10^9/L, and serum amylase is raised at 350 IU/L. An upright chest radiograph demonstrates air under the diaphragm.

3   A 70-year-old woman presents with a 2-day history of colicky central abdominal pain and a 24-hour history of vomiting. On examination there is abdominal distension, visible peristalsis and a midline laparotomy scar. Bowel sounds are tinkling.

4   A 65-year-old woman presents with a 2-day history of constipation, anorexia and pain in her side. On examination, she has a low-grade pyrexia and there is localised tenderness and rebound in the right iliac fossa. Her white blood cell count is 15.0×10^9/L.

5   A 43-year-old man with ankylosing spondylitis presents with a 2-day history of new-onset bloody diarrhoea associated with left-sided abdominal pain. On examination he is pyrexial with left iliac fossa tenderness.

Q₉

a Anterior resection

b Colostomy

c Haemorrhoidectomy

d Hemicolectomy

e High-fibre diet

f Intravenous immunoglobulin

g Loperamide

h Oral steroids

i Topical glyceryl trinitrate ointment (GTN) with anal dilation

j No treatment required

For each of the patients below, choose the **single** most appropriate management from the above list of options. Each option may be used once, more than once or not at all.

1 A 43-year-old man with a history of recurring haemorrhoids continues to suffer from bleeding despite receiving sclerosing therapy.

2 A 37-year-old man has pain and bleeding on defecation. This is his first presentation.

3 A 37-year-old woman who is on mesalazine for her ulcerative colitis presents with unremitting diarrhoea and rectal bleeding. She is noted to have a raised erythrocyte sedimentation rate.

4 A 24-year-old woman following a viral infection was diagnosed as having idiopathic thrombocytopaenia. She presents to the emergency department and complains of multiple bruising and rectal bleeding. She receives an oral prednisolone dose of 30 mg a day. Her haemoglobin is 12.5 g/dL.

5 A 58-year-old man was admitted complaining of abdominal pain. He is found to have rectal carcinoma.

Q10

a Abscess	g Lymphoma
b Aneurysm	h Reactive lymph node
c Folliculitis	i Sebaceous cyst
d Haematoma	j Strangulated femoral
e Inguinal hernia	hernia
f Lipoma	

For each of the patients below, choose the **single** most likely cause of the symptoms from the above list of options. Each option may be used once, more than once or not at all.

1 A 35-year-old man presents for a physical examination arranged by his employer. He explains he has noted an intermittent lump in the right groin for about 8 weeks. It is painless. On examination it is above the inguinal ligament, can be induced by coughing, is reducible and is non-tender.

2 A 40-year-old woman presents with fever, weight loss and malaise for 2 months. Her general practitioner has prescribed her two successive courses of antibiotics for a 'chest infection' to no avail. On examination there is a rubbery 2 cm diameter lump in her right groin and a 1.5 cm diameter lump in her left groin. Said lumps are not tender.

3 A 73-year-old woman with an ulcer on her right lower leg complains about pain in the right groin. On examination there is a tender, warm lump in her right groin.

4 A 72-year-old woman presents with a 2-day history of painful lump in her left groin. On examination there is an exquisitely tender 3 cm mass in her groin.

5 A 52-year-old man presents with a lump in his groin that he thinks is getting bigger. On examination you note a pulsatile mass in his left groin. Past medical history of note, he underwent a coronary angiogram 4 days previously.

Q11

a	Anal fissure	f	Irritable bowel syndrome
b	Angiodysplasia	g	Ischaemic colitis
c	Diverticular disease	h	Rectal carcinoma
d	Duodenal ulcer	i	Sigmoid volvulus
e	Haemorrhoids	j	Ulcerative colitis

For each of the patients below, choose the **single** most likely cause of the symptoms from the above list of options. Each option may be used once, more than once or not at all.

1   A 23-year-old man presents with a history of diarrhoea and weight loss. His bowel habit has changed significantly in recent weeks. He is opening his bowels up to 10 times a day and he notes blood mixed in with his stool.

2   A 31-year-old woman presents with pruritus ani but no pain on defecation. She has also noticed spots of bright-red blood on the toilet paper after defecation.

3   A 53-year-old man presents with left-sided abdominal pain. He explains that it had been intermittent but it is now constant. He has also noted blood in his stool. On examination he is pyrexial and has left iliac fossa tenderness.

4   A 50-year-old man presents with a problem with his back passage. He feels there is still something inside even after he has defecated, and also he is often constipated. He also mentions that he has lost weight unintentionally.

5   A 79-year-old man who has opened his bowels five times over the last 24 hours and passes bright-red blood each time presents. He feels light-headed. On examination you note his pulse rate is 102 beats per minute and his blood pressure is 100/70. He was admitted for a barium enema 1 month previously, which was normal. His haemoglobin on admission then was 12.5 g/dL and now it is 9.5 g/dL.

Q12

a Abdominal aortic aneurysm

b Appendix mass

c Bladder (retention of urine)

d Caecal carcinoma

e Empyema of gallbladder

f Hepatomegaly

g Incisional hernia

h Rectus sheath haematoma

i Sigmoid carcinoma

j Splenomegaly

For each of the patients below, choose the **single** most likely cause of the symptoms from the above list of options. Each option may be used once, more than once or not at all.

1 A 21-year-old man presents with pyrexia, right-sided abdominal pain and anorexia. He explains that he had similar symptoms last week but the pain was more generalised in his abdomen.

2 An 88-year-old man presents after collapsing at his daughter's house. The first vitals recorded are a pulse rate of 110 beats per minute and a blood pressure of 60/30. He is a known sufferer of hypertension and has a 60 pack-year history of smoking.

3 A 63-year-old woman who had a previously perforated duodenal ulcer now presents with a non-tender, central abdominal mass that disappears on lying flat. Her body mass index score is 43.

4 A 25-year-old man who plays professional rugby presents with a mass and pain on his right side. On examination you palpate a firm, non-pulsatile abdominal mass. The pain worsens on movement.

5 A 92-year-old female presented with features of acute small bowel obstruction and a right iliac fossa pain. Of note, the patient has a history of previous appendicectomy.

Q13

a Cryptoorchidism
b Epididymo-orchitis
c Hydrocoele
d Metastases
e Mumps orchitis
f Retractile testis

g Seminoma
h Strangulated indirect inguinal hernia
i Torsion of testis
j Trauma

For each of the patients below, choose the **single** most likely cause of the symptoms from the above list of options. Each option may be used once, more than once or not at all.

1 A 23-year-old man presents with a 6-month history of painful scrotal swelling. On examination there is a hard, smooth swelling of the right testis that is separately palpable. The swelling did not transilluminate and there was no cough impulse.

2 A 16-year-old boy presents with a very sudden onset of severe painful swelling of the scrotum. There was no history of trauma. A very gentle examination reveals a young man with exquisite tenderness of the scrotum.

3 A 77-year-old man presents with a 1-year history of swelling of the scrotum, which has uncharacteristically become painful in the last 4 days. On examination the patient is pyrexial. On examination of his scrotum there is a firm, tender swelling in the left side of the scrotum that extends into the inguinal region. There is no cough impulse.

4 An 18-year-old man who has just started at university presents with a 3-day history of a tender swollen right testicle. Examination reveals tender mandibular swelling and a swollen tender testicle. He is pyrexial.

5 A 52-year-old man presents with fever and a painful testicle. He has recently returned from a conference in South East Asia. On examination you note a tender spermatic cord and testis. He is pyrexial with palpable inguinal lymphadenopathy.

Q14

a Cricothyrotomy

b Endotracheal tube

c Laryngeal mask airway

d Oral airway and oxygen (naso- or oropharyngeal)

e Oxygen facemask with 100% oxygen

f Oxygen facemask with 24% oxygen

g Tracheotomy

h None required

For each of the patients below, choose the **single** most appropriate management from the above list of options. Each option may be used once, more than once or not at all.

1 A 55-year-old man known to suffer from epilepsy arrives in the emergency department after an observed seizure. He is postictal on arrival. On examination you note his breathing is partially obstructed, with an oxygen saturation of 91%.

2 A 19-year-old man suffers a severe head injury after colliding with a lorry while riding a motorcycle. On arrival he has a Glasgow Coma Scale score of 5 and obviously requires an urgent CT scan.

3 A 61-year-old fit man requires an elective knee arthroscopy under general anaesthesia. He has no past medical history and does not suffer from reflux.

4 A 60-year-old woman on your ward has an oxygen saturation of 91% on air. She underwent a laparotomy for small bowel obstruction the previous day. All her other observations are within normal limits. She has no known respiratory disease.

5 A 37-year-old woman is admitted to undergo surgery in the prone position under general anaesthesia.

Q15

a	Aberration of normal development and involution	f	Fat necrosis
		g	Fibroadenoma
		h	Gynaecomastia
b	Benign cyst	i	Mastitis
c	Breast abscess	j	Paget's disease
d	Breast carcinoma		
e	Duct ectasia		

For each of the patients below, choose the **single** most likely cause of the symptoms from the above list of options. Each option may be used once, more than once or not at all.

1 A 40-year-old woman presents with a long history of pain in both breasts. She has kept a diary of the pain and so can tell it is worse just before she menstruates. You find nothing of note on examination.

2 A 19-year-old woman presents with a lump in her right breast. On examination you find a smooth, non-tender lump that is 3 cm in diameter. It is highly mobile.

3 A 30-year-old woman presents with a breast lump 3 months after childbirth. She is still breastfeeding. On examination you find a hard, very red and very tender 4 cm lump at the edge of the left nipple.

4 A 65-year-old woman presents with a breast lump. On examination you find a hard, irregular, non-tender lump that is 3 cm in size. She also explains she has noted a bloody nipple discharge.

5 A 50-year-old woman presents with a tender breast lump. On examination you find a tender, hard 4 cm lump in the left breast. She remembers knocking the breast against a door 6 weeks previously. The woman has a body mass index score of 47.

Q16

a	Arterial ulcer	f	Malignant ulcer
b	Cardiac failure	g	Neuropathic ulcer
c	Cellulitis	h	Pyoderma gangrenosum
d	Deep vein thrombosis	i	Rheumatoid arthritis
e	Lymphadenopathy	j	Venous ulcer

For each of the patients below, choose the **single** most likely cause of the symptoms from the above list of options. Each option may be used once, more than once or not at all.

1   A 44-year-old woman presents with a 4cm chronic painless ulcer on the medial aspect of the lower leg. The ulcer has arisen from an area of skin with scar tissue. The edges of the ulcer are rolled and everted.

2   A 75-year-old woman presents with an ulcer on the anterior aspect of her right shin. She has long-standing hypertension and has had progressive swelling of her legs over the last 4 months. Her main complaint is that the ulcer weeps fluid profusely.

3   A 50-year-old woman presents with a painless ulcer on the plantar aspect of her foot. She is known to be diabetic, with poor control of her blood glucose. She reveals that she has been suffering from a burning feeling on the soles of her feet for the past year.

4   A 70-year-old man presents with an ulcer between the second and third toes on his left foot. He has a past medical history of ischaemic heart disease. The ulcer is associated with pain in the whole foot at night.

5   A 30-year-old woman presents with an ulcer on her mid thigh. She is known to suffer from ulcerative colitis, which is currently in remission. It initially looked like a small insect bite but it has now evolved into a much larger ulcer.

Q₁₇

a Antiembolism stocking

b Check international normalised ratio and continue warfarin

c Embolectomy

d Heparin plus warfarin

e Intravenous heparin

f Observation in hospital

g Reassure and discharge

h Start warfarin therapy

i Subcutaneous low-molecular-weight heparin

j Vena cava filter

For each of the patients below, choose the **single** most appropriate management from the above list of options. Each option may be used once, more than once or not at all.

1 A 25-year-old woman presents with an acutely painful left calf after flying home from Fiji. Ultrasound confirms deep vein thrombosis extending above the popliteal veins. She has recently missed a period and thinks she might be pregnant.

2 A 30-year-old man presents with a pain in his right calf. The pain developed after a game of football. On examination he has marked tenderness but no swelling or erythema. As a precaution you order a Doppler ultrasound scan. This returns as negative.

3 A 50-year-old woman taking non-steroidal anti-inflammatory drugs for osteoarthritis presented with a history of sudden-onset pain behind her right knee leading to pain down the calf. Ultrasound confirms a Baker's cyst. Her mobility is still good.

4 It is 3 a.m. and you are asked to review a 77-year-old woman (who underwent a total hip replacement 3 days ago) with acute chest pain and breathlessness. Electrocardiograph and a chest X-ray show signs of a pulmonary embolism but further imaging is not available until the morning.

5 A 39-year-old woman presents with right leg swelling and increasing pain. She informs you that she is already on warfarin for a deep vein thrombosis in the same leg. Repeat imaging shows thrombus limited to the calf.

Q₁₈

a	Acute prostatitis	f	Chronic prostatitis
b	Advanced prostate cancer	g	Gram-negative septicaemia
c	Bacterial cystitis	h	Hydronephrosis
d	Benign prostatic enlargement	i	Localised prostate disease
e	Bladder calculus	j	Pyelonephritis

For each of the patients below, choose the **single** most likely cause of the symptoms from the above list of options. Each option may be used once, more than once or not at all.

1   A 75-year-old man presents with new-onset back pain. He explains he has just started to experience pain in his back and ribs. Direct questioning reveals he is also suffering from urinary frequency and a poor flow. On digital rectal examination you find a hard prostate.

2   A 60-year-old man presents with bladder pain. He notes he has pain (in the suprapubic area) on standing. He also explains that there is pain on urination and there is sometimes blood in his urine. He has suffered from recurrent urinary infections but is currently dipstick and culture negative.

3   A 65-year-old man presents with a large, painless bladder. He is embarrassed because he sometimes finds himself incontinent of urine at night. Blood results show a raised creatinine level.

4   A 40-year-old man presents with rectal pain. It is a gnawing ache that can be in the rectum or in his perineum. He also reports urinary frequency and dysuria. He has been suffering with these symptoms for 4 months.

5   A 47-year-old man presents with a sudden-onset fever. He adds he is suffering from urinary urgency, frequency and dysuria. Digital rectal examination reveals an exquisitely tender prostate.

Q₁₉

a CT scan
b Diagnostic laparoscopy
c Endoscopy
d Intravenous antibiotics
e Intravenous urogram

f Laparotomy
g Laxatives
h Nasogastric tube
i Serum amylase
j Ultrasound scan

For each of the patients below, choose the **single** most appropriate investigation from the above list of options. Each option may be used once, more than once or not at all.

1 An 18-year-old woman presents with a 1-day history of right iliac fossa pain. On examination you find tenderness and guarding in the right iliac fossa. Digital rectal examination elicits tenderness. She has a negative pregnancy test and there are no menstrual symptoms. Abdominal and pelvic ultrasound scan is normal.

2 A 77-year-old woman presents with a 3-day history of constant left iliac fossa pain. She is pyrexial, with left iliac fossa tenderness. A CT scan demonstrates an inflamed sigmoid colon with numerous diverticula but no perforation.

3 A 45-year-old man presents with sudden-onset epigastric pain that is constant in nature. The pain radiates through to his back. He has had several previous episodes, and he is known to be alcohol dependent.

4 You are asked to review an 80-year-old woman who underwent an operation for a total hip replacement 3 days before. She presents with abdominal distension, colicky pain and profuse vomiting.

5 A 46-year-old woman presents with a 1-week history of constant right upper quadrant pain, radiating around the right side of the chest. On direct questioning she reveals her urine is darker than normal despite drinking more water than usual.

Q₂₀

a Amoxicillin

b Carbimazole

c Excise for biopsy

d Full blood count and heterophile antibody test

e Neck ultrasound scan

f Reassure and send home

g Sialogram

h Technetium thyroid scan

i Thyroxine

j None of the above

For each of the patients below, choose the **single** most appropriate management from the above list of options. Each option may be used once, more than once or not at all.

1 A 47-year-old man presents with an 8-week history of intermittent swelling that occurs below the left side of his jaw during meals but which can occur even if he thinks of food. It disappears overnight. On examination you find a 3 cm, firm lump with no other abnormal findings.

2 A 35-year-old woman presents with anxiety. She notes she is intolerant to heat and has had some weight loss despite a good appetite. On examination you find a resting pulse of 120 beats per minute and she has a fine tremor. She has swelling of the neck in the midline.

3 A 23-year-old woman presents with a 1-week history of a sore throat and fever. On examination you find her submandibular lymph glands are smoothly enlarged and tender.

4 A 37-year-old woman presents with palpitations. She also complains of diarrhoea and weight loss. On examination you find a firm, non-tender lump that is 2 cm in size. This lump moves up and down when the patient swallows.

5 A 50-year-old woman presents with difficulty and pain on swallowing. On examination you find a 10 cm wide mass that appears to be asymmetrical with non-tender nodular masses. Recent blood tests show she is euthyroid.

Answers 1–20

A₁

1 g
This is a straightforward question to ease you into the EMQs. Irritable bowel syndrome is a relapsing and remitting disease characterised by chronic abdominal pain, discomfort, bloating and alteration of bowel habit. There is no known organic cause and it is a diagnosis of exclusion. (Note, it does have a high level of morbidity.)

2 b
Straining at stool and tenesmus (the sensation of not emptying one's rectum) combined with weight loss are red flags for the suspicion of colorectal cancer. Blood and mucus being passed are also important symptoms. That, combined with the patient's age, is a cause for concern.

3 g
Diarrhoea at such a frequency (remember diarrhoea is defined as having three or more loose or liquid bowel movements a day) with signs of systemic interaction should make you think of inflammatory bowel disease. Also note the length of time the patient has suffered with symptoms that correspond with the anaemia.

4 f
The clue is in the backpacking history. It is highly likely that this patient will be suffering from infectious diarrhoea.

5 i
Elective repair is performed in those with symptomatic aneurysms, those that are >5.5 cm, those that are rapidly expanding >1 cm per year and those causing complications (indications developed as a result of the UK Small Aneurysm Trial). One of the known complications of an aortic aneurysm repair is embolism, which can block off the smaller arteries serving the gastrointestinal tract. Other complications include

haemorrhage, renal failure, aorto-duodenal fistula, graft infection, myocardial infarction and multiple organ failure. Note that aneurysms are operated upon at an earlier stage in females than they are in males.

A₂

1 g

Dysphagia (a conscious difficulty in swallowing) can be best divided into oral causes, non-mechanical causes (neurological disorders) and mechanical causes (in the lumen, in the wall or outside the wall). In this case there is an oral cause. A reducible mass on the side of the neck can be the result of a pharyngeal pouch (or Zenker's diverticulum). Risk factors include gastro-oesophageal reflux disease, smoking and excess alcohol consumption.

2 j

A classic presentation of a Hashimoto's thyroiditis. Remember anxiety is not necessarily a diagnosis. It is lymphatic infiltration of the gland due to antibodies produced against thyroglobulin. Thus, as an autoimmune disease (along with type 1 diabetes, Addison's, pernicious anaemia and vitiligo), it is more common in women. The disease usually starts with the patient becoming hyperthyroid and then hypothyroid.

3 c

The man is suffering from a reactive lymph node. However, further investigations must be planned if it persists and becomes painless, as it could be lymphadenopathy due to Hodgkin's disease.

4 e

A young man with neck and scrotal swelling invariably has mumps, which is a variant of parotitis. Males past puberty who develop mumps have a 20% risk of orchitis. It is important to recognise mumps in an older male patient because of the significant risk to future fertility.

5 h

The patient has a thyroglossal cyst, which occurs if remnants of the thyroglossal duct persist. They are smooth and round and they are found in the midline. Classically the lump will move upwards when a patient swallows. Treatment is excision of the lump. After observation, on examination of the thyroid (unless specifically asked to start at the gland), start with the hands. Look for any swellings, goitre, scars or asymmetry. Then look at the hands for thyroid acropachy and palmar erythema while feeling for temperature and the pulse rate. Then move onto the eyes. Make a point of looking for exophthalmos, proptosis and lid lag. Then stand in front of the patient and ask him or her to swallow – this helps determine whether a lump moves on swallowing. Then ask the patient to protrude the tongue, specifically looking for a thyroglossal cyst. Then standing behind the patient, palpate each lobe of the thyroid separately. Ask the patient to sip water and hold it in his or her mouth until you ask them to swallow – note whether the lump moves or not. Examine the mass as you would for any other lump. Palpate for local lymph nodes. Feel for tracheal deviation. Percuss the sternum to ensure no retrosternal thyroid (remember the thyroid can extend well behind the sternum) and listen for a bruit. Ask the patient to stand (looking for proximal myopathy).

A3

1 h

This is the classic presentation of a pancreatic pseudocyst, and this is a complication of acute pancreatitis. They account for 75% of all pancreatic masses. They are known as pseudocysts, as they are lined with granulation tissue as opposed to epithelium. After an episode of acute pancreatitis there is an extravasation of pancreatic enzymes, which digest the adjoining tissue. Many collections resolve on their own, but others become organised and become walled off with the layer of granulation tissue and fibrosis.

2 b

Normally the two sides of the rectus abdominis muscle are joined at the linea alba. In pregnant or post-partum women the growing uterus stretches the rectus abdominis. Risk factors include pregnancy over the age of 35, high birthweight of the child and multiple-birth pregnancies. Treatment is primarily conservative and involves physiotherapy. Surgery is required in serious cases.

3 i

Around 50% of all patients with glandular fever (infectious mononucleosis) develop an enlarged spleen in the first few weeks after infection. While splenic rupture is rare, it is important to inform your patient of the risks.

4 g

Where a child presents with massive haematemesis and accompanying splenomegaly, oesophageal varices should always be very high up on the differential. The child is likely to be suffering from portal hypertension (i.e. the portal venous pressure is 10–12 mmHg higher than in the inferior vena cava). If the patient is known to suffer from oesophageal varices, prophylactic sclerotherapy may be offered. The successful treatment of the portal hypertension depends upon the cause.

5 g

This is the classic emergency presentation of oesophageal varices in an adult. From 5% to 10% of upper gastrointestinal bleeds are caused by oesophageal varices. This patient must be treated as an emergency. Protect the airway and insert two large-bore cannulae while taking blood for crossmatch; start high-flow oxygen; give intravenous colloid quickly and then blood, aiming for a haemoglobin >10 g/dL. Catheterise and monitor urine output. Correctly clotting abnormalities and set up central venous pressure line to guide fluid replacement. Note, the indications for surgery are severe bleeding, a Rockall score >6, re-bleeding, active bleeding during oesophagogastroduodenoscopy and continuing bleeding after transfusion.

A4

1 g

Because of the mechanism of a seizure, most shoulder dislocations are posterior. Note that most shoulder dislocations, not caused by a seizure (up to 98%) are anterior. They are generally caused by the shoulder being held in internal rotation and adduction. Attempted abduction and external rotation are painful. The arm cannot be externally rotated into a neutral position. The anteroposterior view on radiograph of the head of the humerus may resemble a light bulb because of rotation – the 'light bulb' sign.

2 i

A twisting mechanism of injury is likely to cause a spiral fracture when part of the bone is unable to move (e.g. when it is strapped in a ski boot). Note that over the anterior and medial tibia, the skin and subcutaneous tissue is very thin and thus a great number of tibial fractures are open fractures.

3 j

This is a common fracture in children under the age of 10 years. The elbow hyperextends (due to laxity of the ligaments) when a child tries to catch him- or herself during a fall, and the olecranon process is forced again the weaker metaphyseal bone of the distal humerus. This produces the common extension-type injury where the distal fragment is displaced posteriorly.

4 f

Also known as a stress fracture, in runners a March fracture most often occurs at the metatarsal neck. It occurs following prolonged stress, and the history of direct trauma is very rare. Those with pes cavus are more susceptible to such fractures.

5 h

This is a typical history and presentation of a scaphoid fracture. Note the complications of scaphoid injuries include non-union, avascular necrosis and arthritis.

A5

1 j

While the patient has no stridor, he is having difficulty in swallowing and talking. Dysphagia, stridor, dysphonia or an expanding neck haematoma are all indications to explore a penetrating neck wound, despite its apparent superficiality. It should be explored in theatre as soon as possible.

2 i

Inability to flex the tip of a middle finger indicates there is an injury to the flexor digitorum profundus tendon.

3 a

This woman is suffering from a tension pneumothorax. Prompt decompression is vital, as this is an emergency; there is no time to confirm this with a chest radiograph. Either a chest tube (closed thoracostomy tube drainage) must be inserted or a large-bore cannula can be inserted in the second intercostal space in the midclavicular line.

However, the second method only buys time until a chest drain can be inserted.

4 j

This patient may have compromised arterial blood flow distal to the stab wound and thus is at risk of ischaemia. This wound must be explored immediately in theatre. If possible, an angiogram of the vessels can be performed simultaneously to ascertain the level of damage. Remember the 6 Ps of an ischaemic limb are pallor, pulselessness, paresthesia, pain, paralysis and perishingly cold. It takes as little as 4 hours for limb loss to occur.

5 j

This is a traumatic diaphragmatic hernia. These are commonly associated with deceleration injuries. It is often a sign of severe trauma and thus often presents with other fractures.

A6

1 d

Over-the-counter non-steroidal anti-inflammatory drugs are associated with an increased risk of developing a peptic ulcer. In this case it is a gastric ulcer, as the pain increases on eating. It is now bleeding enough to cause melaena. Duodenal ulcers are relieved by food but are painful at night.

2 b

Crohn's disease has a higher incidence and prevalence in the Ashkenazi Jewish population. This implies a genetic component, but while multiple genes have been implicated, there is no consensus as to the cause.

3 e

A Mallory–Weiss tear is due to forceful vomiting leading to a tear of the mucosa at the gastro-oesophageal junction. The tear involves the mucosa and the submucosa but not the muscular layer (note, this is in contrast to Boerhaave's syndrome). Treatment is usually supportive, although it is an arterial bleed so cauterisation may be required.

4 g

This man is presenting with oesophageal cancer. Smoking is one of the leading causes. The tumour is obviously bleeding to cause melaena.

Note, two-thirds of tumours will be inoperable at time of discovery. The overall 5-year survival rate is 5%.

5 f

This is a classic presentation of a Meckel's diverticulum. This diverticulum is a remnant of the vitellointestinal duct. Remember the rule of 2s: 2% of the population, 2 feet proximal to the ileocaecal valve, 2 inches in length, most common presentation at 2 years of age, 2:1 male to female ratio and there are two common types of ectopic tissue (gastric and pancreatic). Haemorrhage is the most likely complication. Other complications include intestinal obstruction and neoplasia.

A7

1 e

A gastroscopy is to exclude gastric cancer. However, considering the unintentional weight loss and the sense of fullness, it is likely that this patient is suffering from the disease.

2 j

The history implies a ruptured abdominal aortic aneurysm. There is a 100% mortality rate without surgery and a 50%–75% mortality rate with surgery. The fact the patient is still alive implies it was a retroperitoneal rupture. The pressure of the haematoma prevents the blood volume being depleted. Time is of the essence. Insert two large-bore cannulae while taking bloods for a full blood count, urea and electrolytes, clotting, liver function tests and crossmatch for 10 units. The patient may well be hypotensive but on this occasion aggressive fluid resuscitation may blow the tamponade of the haematoma. Thus permissive hypotension is instilled where the systolic blood pressure does not go higher than 80 mmHg. Call for senior help and inform the anaesthetists. The patient is then sent to theatre (after imaging if stable enough) for the aorta to be cross-clamped proximal to the rupture for the haemorrhage to be controlled.

3 g

This woman is suffering from irritable bowel syndrome. However, she may be referred for further investigation if there is unintentional weight loss, rectal bleeding, anaemia, abdominal or rectal masses, raised inflammatory markers, family history of bowel or ovarian cancer, or if the patient is aged over 60 and experiences a change of bowel habit for more than 6 weeks.

4   j

This patient is likely to be suffering from cholecystitis. The pain is in the right upper quadrant and it radiates to the back at around T7. There is marked tenderness in the right hypochondrium and Murphy's sign may be present. Place two fingers over the right upper quadrant under the costal margin and ask the patient to breathe in; listen for a wince or gasp (arrest of breathing) with pain as the gallbladder moves and hits the fingers. However, this must be negative on the left-hand side and it is not a very accurate sign. Ultrasound should confirm the presence of gallstones. Remember the 5 Fs of gallstones: fair, fat, forty, fertile and female.

5   i

This appears to be an infective diarrhoea. Checking for pathogens in the stool is the appropriate course of action.

A8

1   d

This man is likely to be suffering from diverticulitis. Admission should be arranged when pain cannot be controlled with simple analgesia, good hydration is difficult, if there is significant co-morbidity or if there are complications associated with perforation. Co-amoxiclav and metronidazole are typical antibiotics used to treat the supposed infection.

2   g

A perforated peptic ulcer is suggested here because of the air under the diaphragm and other symptoms. A normal amylase level is between 23 and 85 IU/L. Note, the causes of hyperamylasaemia include acute pancreatitis (usually five times the high end of normal), pancreatic cancer, cholecystitis, severe gastroenteritis, bowel obstruction, pancreatic or bile duct blockage and ectopic pregnancy rupture.

3   i

The symptoms suggest a small bowel obstruction. In developed countries, the commonest cause of bowel obstruction is adhesions. This patient has a laparotomy scar and is at risk of developing adhesions. To differentiate clinically between a small and a large bowel obstruction, note that central colicky pain is a symptom of a small bowel obstruction. Intuitively, vomiting occurs with small bowel obstructions (the contents of the vomitus will be as follows. Pre small bowel no bile, bilious distal to the ampulla of Vater and faeculent is most distal). Large bowel obstructions tend to cause constipation of faeces and flatus and distension. On radiograph the small bowel is visible with lines crossing the entire section of bowel (valvulae conniventes), and the large bowel is more peripheral with lines that only partially cross the bowel (haustra).

4 c

This patient is suffering from appendicitis. Note, there is a bimodal distribution for appendicitis – the first peak is in the second-third decade and the second peak is in later life. Surgery is usually indicated.

5 j

Ankylosing spondylitis is associated with ulcerative colitis. There is also a strong association with the surface antigen human leukocyte antigen B27.

A9

1 c

If sclerosing therapy is ineffective then a surgical option is preferred. A haemorrhoidectomy involves excision and ligation of the vascular pedicles. Remember the patient will need preoperative bowel preparation and he or she will need to be sent home with laxatives post-operatively. Complications of the haemorrhoidectomy include sphincter damage.

2 e

This patient is suffering from haemorrhoids. Haemorrhoids tend to occur at the positions 3, 7 and 11 o'clock if the patient is viewed in the lithotomy position. This is because three major arteries that enter the anal canal at these three points feed the vascular plexuses within the anal cushions that become engorged and disrupted. Remember these are not varicose veins of the anus. Conservative treatment includes a high-fibre diet, stopping straining when passing stools and good anal hygiene.

3 h

This patient is suffering from an acute attack – this is where there are more than six motions a day of bloody diarrhoea with systemic symptoms. The immediate treatment for an attack includes intravenous access, as the patient is likely to be fluid depleted, putting the patient nil by mouth, commencement of steroid therapy, the use of antibiotics if there is a perforation or peritonitis, and immunosuppression (with infliximab).

4 f

Rectal and other gastrointestinal bleeding is a serious and possibly fatal complication of idiopathic thrombocytopenic purpura. Thus this is an emergency and the patient requires intravenous immunoglobulin. It is extremely expensive but it can increase the platelet count and reduce the bleeding risk further. Other treatments to consider are mycophenolate mofetil and azathioprine, thrombopoietin receptor agonists and, in a very grave situation, platelet transfusion.

5 a

An anterior resection is possible with tumours up to 4 cm from the anal verge. An anastomosis is created between the rectal stump and the descending colon and no colostomy is required. If the tumour is within 4 cm of the anal verge an abdominoperineal resection is performed. This requires a permanent colostomy because of the removal of the anus. Note, if it is thought the tumour has spread locally, a total mesenteric excision is undertaken. This includes the removal of the mesentery of the rectum during an anterior resection to decrease the incidence of local occurrence. Rectal carcinoma extends radially into the surrounding mesentery.

A10

1 e

This man is suffering from an inguinal hernia. While it can be difficult to determine the type of hernia, it appears this is an indirect inguinal hernia, as it is not controlled by coughing. The only definitive way to determine the type of inguinal hernia is in theatre. If the defect is medial to the inferior epigastric vessels it is direct, and if it is lateral, it is indirect.

2 g

Persistent, rubbery, non-tender lymph nodes are a red flag for lymphoma. As these are found in the groin it is likely she could be suffering from stage I Hodgkin's lymphoma. Stage I is the involvement of a single lymph node region, usually the cervical region or a single extralymphatic site; stage II is the involvement of two or more lymph node regions on the same side of the diaphragm or of one lymph node region and a contiguous extralymphatic site; stage III is involvement of lymph node regions on both sides of the diaphragm, which may include the spleen and/or limited contiguous extralymphatic organ or site; and stage IV is disseminated involvement of one or more extralymphatic organs. Management is complicated and depends upon many factors and local protocols.

3 h

This patient is suffering from a reactive lymph node because of the ulcer on her leg. This could be due to infection from cellulitis. A swab should be taken to see if the area is indeed infected. Likely organisms to be implicated are *Staphylococcus* spp.

4 j

This patient is suffering from a strangulated femoral hernia. On examination it can be differentiated from an inguinal hernia because it lies below and lateral to the pubic tubercle. Approximately 50% of femoral hernias present as an emergency, because the walls of the femoral canal are quite rigid and the neck of the canal is narrow.

5 b

Technically this is a pseudoaneurysm and is usually iatrogenic, because of the femoral artery being the vessel of choice for most endovascular arterial interventions. Ultrasound-guided thrombin injections are thought to be the most efficacious in treating the defect. There may be an accompanying haematoma and thus d may also be a correct answer.

A11

1 j

This is a classic presentation of ulcerative colitis. Remember this is a relapsing and remitting disease that always involves the rectum and spreads proximally. It can also involve the terminal ileum via backwash ileitis. There is an association with non-smokers. Fifteen per cent develop extensive disease and 20% develop pancolitis.

2 e

Bright-red blood is indicative of haemorrhoids. First-degree haemorrhoids do not prolapse out of the anal canal and are therefore not palpable. Second-degree haemorrhoids prolapse out of the anus on defecation and reduce spontaneously. Third-degree haemorrhoids prolapse and remain outside the rectum unless repositioned manually. Fourth-degree haemorrhoids remain persistently prolapsed. Large piles may thrombose if their venous return is obstructed by sphincter tone and they then become painful and are known as strangulated.

3 c

This patient is suffering from diverticular disease, which is defined as diverticula with symptoms. Diverticula are outpouchings of the colonic wall and they usually result from the herniation of the mucosa through the muscular layer due to the penetration of mesenteric vessels. They are most common in the sigmoid colon. Diverticulosis is the asymptomatic presence of diverticula; diverticulitis is the evidence of diverticular inflammation with or without localised symptoms or signs. Remember Saint's triad of a hiatus hernia, diverticular disease and cholelithiasis, which is indicative of a Western lifestyle.

4 h

This patient has rectal carcinoma. Staging of the disease is via the Dukes classification. Dukes A is where the tumour is confined to the bowel wall; prognosis is 85% at 5 years if adequately resected. Dukes B is where the tumour has infiltrated the bowel wall but there is no lymph node involvement and there is a 60% 5-year survival rate. Dukes C involves lymph nodes with a 30% chance of survival. Dukes D, an added stage, is where there are distant metastases with a poor survival rate of 5% at 5 years.

5 b

Angiodysplasia is a small vascular malformation of the gastrointestinal system. It is a cause of unexplained gastrointestinal bleeding. The lesions are often multiple and most frequently occur in the ascending colon and the caecum.

A₁₂

1 b

This patient is suffering from appendicitis. An inflammation of the vermiform appendix leads to changes such as oedema through to ischaemia and perforation. There is a maximal incidence in childhood because of the narrow neck of the appendix. The majority of cases are due to obstruction with a faecolith. The classic history (which occurs in 50% of cases) is as follows: there is a gradual onset of central, colicky abdominal pain and this pain then shifts to the right iliac fossa; the visceral pain now has become somatic, and this pain is worse on movement; there is nausea with or with vomiting, and there is a low-grade fever and anorexia. It is prudent to exclude ectopic pregnancy. There is guarding and rebound tenderness, usually over McBurney's point, and pain can be felt on per rectum examination, which can mean a retrocaecal appendix.

2 a

The man is suffering from a ruptured abdominal aortic aneurysm. The classic triad of pain in the flank or back, hypotension and a pulsatile abdominal mass is only present in 50% of cases. Abdominal pain is the most frequent symptom, followed by back pain, syncope and vomiting.

3 g

An incisional hernia is a hernia that occurs through a previously made incision in the abdominal wall. If pain is felt, it is felt over the defect and is greatest at the fascial margins. The presence of an irreducible hernia requires a prompt surgical referral, and if there is sharp pain or signs of peritonitis, urgent surgical referral is necessary. Most incisional defects are repaired with mesh.

4 h

A rectus sheath haematoma is the result of bleeding into the rectus sheath from the superior or inferior epigastric vessels or from a direct tear of the sheath itself. When derived from trauma, the initial incident could be quite minor. However, tight contraction of the recti in anticipation of the blow predisposes to rectus sheath haematoma formation.

5 d

A common way for caecal carcinoma to present is through small bowel obstruction. Note that the symptoms can clinically mimic appendicitis.

A₁₃

1 g

Seminomas present more often than teratomas in older males. They arise from the germinal cells in the testes. They are solid and slow growing. They are very radiosensitive and thus have a 5-year survival rate of 90%. Of note, if there are metastases on discovery of the lump there will be a raised placental alkaline phosphatase.

2 i

Exquisite unilateral pain and swelling of the scrotum is likely to be caused by torsion of the testes. This is a surgical emergency. They may also present with lower abdominal pain (testicles are innervated at the level of T10). The testicle will be hot and swollen. It should also be lying transversely. The cord in torsion may also be palpable (if they let you palpate it!). There is up to a 6-hour window from the onset of pain in which the testicle is still salvageable. In this case, inform a senior colleague, place the patient nil by mouth, gain intravenous access and take bloods for a full blood count, urea and electrolytes, clotting and group and save, and give analgesia. There is not time for a diagnostic ultrasound scan. Remember to gain consent for exploration of the testis plus or minus orchiectomy and to gain consent for fixing of the contralateral side.

3 h

Up to 15% of patients with hernias will present as an emergency in this way. They are more common on the right side. The contents of the inguinal canal in a male is as follows: cremasteric fascia and the internal spermatic fascia; the spermatic cord, the vas deferens and lymphatics, arteries to the vas deferens, cremaster and the testes; the pampiniform plexus and the genital branch of the genitofemoral nerve; finally, the ilioinguinal nerve passes through the superficial ring to descend into the scrotum, but is not technically part of the inguinal canal. Note that in the female it is the round ligament of the uterus and the ilioinguinal nerve.

4 e

Mumps leading to orchitis in adult males occurs in approximately 30% of cases. This is a painful and dangerous complication. Half of these infections lead to testicular atrophy with the potential for infertility.

5 b

Epididymo-orchitis is the commonest cause of acute scrotal pain. However, the most important differential diagnosis that should be excluded is testicular torsion. If epididymo-orchitis is thought to be due to a sexually transmitted infection, including gonorrhoea, treat it without waiting for test results with oral doxycycline 100 mg twice daily for 10–14 days, plus a single dose of intramuscular ceftriaxone 500 mg and refer to a sexual health clinic for follow-up.

A₁₄

1 d

This patient is breathing but needs help, as his oxygen saturation is certainly lower than 100%. He is maintaining his own airway and thus a naso- or oropharyngeal airway is indicated.

2 b

A Glasgow Coma Scale score of less than 8 indicates the patient requires tracheal intubation to protect his airway and prevent aspiration.

3 c

This patient is otherwise healthy and thus the less invasive laryngeal mask airway can be used. If it had not required general anaesthesia, a regional block may have been considered.

4 e

This woman may be experiencing a complication of her surgery. Thus she should be given a face mask with 100% oxygen before further examination and tests are done. Note, if an arterial blood gas on air is required then the patient should have been off face mask oxygen for at least 10 minutes.

5 b

Because the patient needs to be in the prone position, tracheal intubation is required. Laryngeal mask airways have been used in this situation; however, intraoperative access is more difficult and thus tracheal tubing is preferred.

A15

1 a

Aberration of normal development and involution is an umbrella term for a number of conditions affecting women (usually between the ages of 30 and 50 years) and thus hormone related. It includes fibrosis, adenosis, cyst formation, epitheliosis and papillomatosis. However, if lumps are detected, neoplasia should be first ruled out. Usually reassurance and a good bra are enough to console the patient. Analgesia and evening primrose oil are also helpful. (Although, do note the many interactions with medications that evening primrose oil has.) Other drugs that can be used include danazol (but has androgenic side effects) or bromocriptine (which is a dopamine agonist and thus decreases prolactin).

2 g

Fibroadenomas (breast mice) account for 20% of breast masses. They are firm, smooth and mobile. A third regress, a third stay the same and a third increase in size. If they are larger than 5 cm they are usually excised. Malignant change is very rare.

3 i

Bacteria are usually the cause of acute mastitis. It is extremely painful. Cultures should be taken, and the mother should be given analgesia and antibiotics and be advised to rest. Since this is invariably staphylococcal infection, flucloxacillin is indicated.

4 d

This patient is likely to be suffering from breast cancer. The most important signs to note are a firm, irregular and painless lump (usually in the upper outer quadrant), bloody nipple discharge, nipple retraction, axillary lymph nodes, Paget's disease, periductal oedema (peau d'orange), signs of metastasis and puckering or tethering due to contraction of the ligaments of Astley Cooper. The patient undergoes a triple assessment: (i) examination; (ii) imaging, usually ultrasound scan (or radiograph); and (iii) needle biopsy. It is staged with the TMN classification of malignant tumours.

5 f

Fat necrosis occurs after trauma (which can be very minor) because of trauma fibrosis and calcification. Such lumps can mimic a neoplastic mass. Lipase releases fatty acids from triglycerides that combine with calcium.

A₁₆

1 f

This is likely to be a Marjolin's ulcer, an aggressive squamous cell carcinoma that occurs in scarred skin. It grows slowly and is painless (no nerve tissue), and there is an absence of lymphatic spread because of local destruction. Treatment is wide excision of the lesion.

2 e

The lymphoedema may be due to heart failure or another medical course and thus a secondary cause. Primary lymphoedema is rare. Note, the lymphoedematous limb is particularly prone to sepsis and thus patients should be made aware of the importance of hygiene. Before palpating such a limb, do remember to ask about pain. Gentle palpation will distinguish between pitting and non-pitting oedema.

3 g

A diabetic neuropathy is the main clue here. Progressive loss of light touch and vibration (and some motor) sense because of the mixed nerve neuropathy can lead to unnoticed wounds in the feet. These neuropathic changes can occur even with good glucose control.

4 a

These are colloquially known as kissing ulcers (although don't confuse them with the genital sort!). Arterial ulcers (note the ischaemic heart disease) start with irregular edges and then become the punched-out ulcer. The base contains greyish granulation tissue. Nocturnal pain is common, especially when lying down; hanging the leg out of bed relieves this pain. Eighty per cent of ulcers can be managed in primary care; however, you should refer when the Ankle Brachial Pressure Index value is less than 0.8 and urgently if it is less than 0.5. Also refer if there is a suspicion of malignancy or if it is associated with systemic vasculitis.

5 h

Ulcerative colitis is associated with pyoderma gangrenosum. It has a purulent surface and a blue-black edge. It classically begins as nodules, which break down into a rapidly enlarging ulcer.

A17

1 i

She has a proven deep vein thrombosis and is therefore at risk of this causing a pulmonary embolism. Obviously, warfarin would be contraindicated because of the possibility of pregnancy. Deep vein thromboses that extend further that the popliteal veins need to be treated, thus low-molecular-weight heparin is used. Low-molecular-weight heparin does not cross the placenta and nor does it pass into breast milk. (Note, however, it is possible to use warfarin after childbirth.) Problems associated with low-molecular-weight heparin include its long half-life, it is not to be used with epidural anaesthesia, protamine sulphate (the antidote) is less effective, it is difficult to monitor accurately and it is more expensive.

2 g

This is most likely to be a muscular strain and the man should be treated with RICE (rest, ice, compression and elevation).

3 g

This patient is suffering from a Baker's cyst, which is synovial swelling behind the knee – not a true cyst but a dilatation of the gastrocnemius semimembranosus bursa. In adults they are usually secondary to degenerative and inflammatory arthritis, meniscal tears and anterior cruciate ligament damage. Management includes reassurance, as rest and simple analgesia should help with the pain and the cyst should resolve on its own. You should also seek to optimise the management of the osteoarthritis, which may include aspiration of the joint and a corticosteroid injection. Surgery is not usually helpful in those with severe osteoarthritis.

4 e

Heparin should be given to patients with intermediate or high clinical probability before imaging. Unfractionated heparin should be considered as a first-dose bolus, in massive pulmonary embolism or where rapid reversal of effect may be needed. Otherwise, low-molecular-weight heparin should be considered as preferable to unfractionated heparin, having equal efficacy and safety and being easier to use. The target international normalised ratio should be 2.0–3.0; when this is achieved, heparin can be discontinued. Senior help should be sought for this case.

5   b

It is prudent to check this woman's international normalised ratio. Remember, adequate anti-coagulation is important to avoid the development of post-thrombotic syndrome. This develops after a deep vein thrombosis because of damage to the deep veins and their valves. It can cause minor problems (skin changes) or major problems (chronic pain and swelling and ulceration).

Note, because of the unreliability of clinical features, many use Wells' diagnostic algorithm.

Score one point for each of the following:

- active cancer
- paralysis or plaster immobilisation of the legs
- recently bedridden for 3 days or more, or major surgery within the previous 12 weeks, requiring general or regional anaesthesia
- localised tenderness along the distribution of the deep venous system (such as the back of the calf)
- entire leg is swollen
- calf swelling by more than 3 cm compared with the asymptomatic leg (measured 10 cm below the tibial tuberosity)
- pitting oedema confined to the symptomatic leg
- collateral superficial veins (not varicose veins)
- previously documented deep vein thrombosis.

Subtract two points if an alternative cause is considered at least as likely as deep vein thrombosis. The risk of deep vein thrombosis is likely if the score is two or more, and unlikely if the score is one or less.

A18

1   a

Prostate cancer is the most common cancer in men and the third most common cause of cancer death in the Western world in men. It is an androgen-driven cancer, adenocarcinoma in type and tends to manifest in the outer zone of the gland (in contrast to benign prostatic hyperplasia) and then infiltrates the whole of the gland to leave it hard. If it has spread to the bones, the lesions are osteosclerotic and therefore appear denser than bone on radiograph. The Gleason score for the different stages of the cancer combines information taken from the digital rectal exam, an ultrasound scan of the prostate and liver, a bone scan and the prostate-specific antigen test.

2 d

This man is suffering from bladder calculi. They are usually associated with urinary stasis. His history of urinary infection increases the risk of stone formation. (Note, long-standing untreated bladder calculi are associated with squamous cell carcinoma.) Small stones can be removed using lithotripsy; larger stones require open surgery.

3 d

This is the common presentation of benign prostatic hyperplasia, a benign nodular or diffuse proliferation of the musculofibrous and glandular layers of the prostate. Symptoms can be acute because of urinary obstruction or more commonly are due to detrusor instability leading to the following urinary symptoms: nocturia, urinary frequency, post-micturition dribbling, poor stream, strangury (painful, frequent urination of small volumes that are expelled slowly only by straining and despite urgency, usually with the sensation of incomplete emptying – tenesmus for the bladder), straining, hesitancy and overflow incontinence.

4 f

This patient is suffering from chronic prostatitis, which can severely reduce quality of life. (However, there is no obviously inflammatory pathology associated with the disease.) Patients with chronic prostatitis also suffer from sexual dysfunction and may be embarrassed to talk about the subject. Management includes explaining this is not cancer or a sexually transmitted infection. Refer to urology, who may start a trial for an alpha blocker.

5 a

This man is suffering from acute prostatitis, a non-sexually transmitted bacterial infection of the prostate. Take a urine sample for microscopy, culture and sensitivity and start ciprofloxacin 500 mg twice daily for 28 days. After 48 hours ensure the appropriate antibiotic is being used.

A₁₉

1 b

This patient is most likely suffering from appendicitis. Right iliac fossa pain accounts for half of all cases of acute abdominal pain, and in only half of those suspected to have appendicitis is the preoperative diagnosis correct. Note, causes of right iliac fossa include appendicitis, urinary tract infection, non-specific abdominal pain, pelvic inflammatory disease, renal colic, ectopic pregnancy and constipation. Remember the bimodal distribution for appendicitis – the second peak is in later life.

2 d

This patient appears to be suffering from acute diverticulitis. Admission should be arranged when pain cannot be controlled with simple analgesia, when good hydration is difficult, if there is significant co-morbidity or if there are complications associated with perforation. Co-amoxiclav and metronidazole are typical antibiotics used.

3 i

This patient appears to be suffering from acute pancreatitis. Aetiology includes (I GET SMASHED) Idiopathic, Gallstones, Ethanol, Trauma, Steroids, Metabolic disorders, Autoimmune disorders, Scorpion venom (this is extremely rare! Never say this first!), Hypercalcaemia, hyperlipidaemia and hypothermia, Endoscopic retrograde cholangiopancreatography and Drugs. Initial treatment includes pain relief, intravenous fluids, antibiotics if indicated, supplementary oxygen and early nutritional support.

4 h

This patient appears to be suffering from Ogilvie's syndrome, a relatively rare condition where there is an acute intestinal pseudo-obstruction associated with massive dilatation of the colon (usually the caecum). It is associated with total joint replacement surgery and coronary artery bypass grafting. Treatment includes a nasogastric tube to help decompress the stomach, but colonoscopic decompression may be required. Neostigmine has been used, but in this patient group co-morbidities are rife. Gastrografin enemas have been found to be helpful in the decompression.

5 j

This woman is suffering from cholecystitis; an ultrasound scan should reveal gallstones in the gallbladder and perhaps some in the biliary tree leading to an obstructive jaundice. Treatment includes intravenous fluids, antibiotics and analgesia, and assessment for a cholecystectomy.

A20

1 g

This patient is suffering from a blocked salivary duct. It is the submandibular duct (Wharton's duct) in 90% of cases. A sialogram shows 80% of radiopaque calculi. Management includes removal of the stone by massaging the gland; lemon drops can induce salivation to help clear the stone; maintain good hydration and avoid diuretics. Consider ear, nose and throat referral if the stone does not pass in a week.

2 b

This patient is suffering from hyperthyroidism. If the physical symptoms are overt, consider also prescribing a beta blocker, to relieve the adrenergic symptoms.

3 d

This patient may be suffering from infectious mononucleosis. The most common virus to cause this is the Epstein–Barr virus, but it can also be attributed to cytomegalovirus. Note, if the first heterophile antibody test (Paul–Bunnell ovine red blood cells or Monospot equine red blood cells) comes back negative this does not discount infectious mononucleosis. Positivity increases in the first 6 weeks of the illness (a 25% false-negative rate in the first week, 10% in the second and 5% in the third). Treatment is usually supportive (do not give ampicillin or amoxicillin, as it can lead to an itchy maculopapular rash). Also, splenomegaly may persist for up to 8 weeks.

4 h

This patient has symptoms of an overactive thyroid, but with a painless nodular lump, cancer should be suspected. Papillary carcinomas are the most common and account for up to 70% of thyroid cancers. They are three times more common in women. They tend to spread locally and metastases are commonly found in the lung and bone.

5 j

This non-toxic goitre appears to have extended posteriorly to cause dysphagia. Note recent accelerated growth should raise suspicion of malignancy. Treatment is considered when there is growth of the entire goitre, compressive symptoms or thyrotoxicosis. Treatment includes thyroidectomy, radioactive iodine therapy and T4 (levothyroxine) therapy.

Index

abdomen, rigid and guarded (Q) 93, *(A) 100*

abdominal aortic aneurysm (Q) 39, *(A) 44*
  leaking (Q) 40, *(A) 45*; (Q) 41, *(A) 46*
  ruptured (Q) 112, *(A) 133*; (Q) 118, *(A) 139*

abdominal distension (Q) 6, *(A) 13*; (Q) 125, *(A) 147*

abdominal mass
  central (Q) 118, *(A) 139*
  midline (Q) 108, *(A) 129*

abdominal pain
  central (Q) 112, *(A) 133*
  colicky (Q) 7, *(A) 14*; (Q) 53, *(A) 56*; (Q) 114, *(A) 134–5*
  diffuse (Q) 110, *(A) 132*; (Q) 111, *(A) 132–3*
  left-sided (Q) 117, *(A) 138*
  right-sided (Q) 118, *(A) 139*
  sudden (Q) 40, *(A) 45*
  upper (Q) 108, *(A) 129*

abdominal X-ray
  and gallstones (Q) 22, *(A) 26*
  plain (Q) 6, *(A) 13–14*

achalasia (Q) 3, *(A) 12*

Achilles tendon rupture (Q) 72, *(A) 75*

acoustic neuroma (Q) 77, *(A) 81*

adhesions (Q) 7, *(A) 14*

adrenaline, nebulised (Q) 79, *(A) 81*

alcohol, and carcinomas (Q) 4, *(A) 12*

alpha-adrenergic antagonist (Q) 59, *(A) 64*

amitriptyline (Q) 60, *(A) 65*

amniotic fluid embolism (Q) 38, *(A) 44*

anatomical snuffbox (Q) 70, *(A) 75*; (Q) 109, *(A) 131*

aneurysm, iatrogenic (Q) 116, *(A) 137*

angiodysplasia (Q) 117, *(A) 138*

angular stomatitis (Q) 3, *(A) 12*

ankylosing spondylitis (Q) 114, *(A) 135*

anterior resection (Q) 115, *(A) 136*

antibiotics
  and breast disorders (Q) 29, *(A) 35*; (Q) 32, *(A) 36*
  intravenous (Q) 68, *(A) 74*

aortic aneurysm, elective repair (Q) 106, *(A) 127–8*

APC (adenomatous polyposis coli) (Q) 10, *(A) 16*

appendicitis (Q) 114, *(A) 135*; (Q) 118, *(A) 139*; (Q) 125, *(A) 147*

arterial insufficiency, early (Q) 37, *(A) 44*

arterial ulcers (Q) 122, *(A) 143*

arthritis, septic (Q) 67, *(A) 74*

back pain (Q) 69, *(A) 75*; (Q) 124, *(A) 145–6*

Baker's cyst (Q) 123, *(A) 144*

balloon dilatation (Q) 9, *(A) 15*

barium swallow (Q) 7, *(A) 14*

Barrett's oesophagus (Q) 5, *(A) 13*

basal skull fracture (Q) 89, *(A) 99*

Beck's triad (Q) 96, *(A) 101*

benign prostatic hyperplasia (Q) 58–9, *(A) 64*; (Q) 124, *(A) 146*

bile duct, stones in (Q) 21, *(A) 25*

bladder calculi (Q) 124, *(A) 146*

bladder outflow obstruction (Q) 59, *(A) 64*

blood count
    and mononucleosis (Q) 126,
      (A) 148
    and nosebleed (Q) 84, (A) 87
branchial cyst (Q) 83, (A) 87
breast cancer (Q) 121, (A) 142
    and ductal carcinoma in situ
      (Q) 28, (A) 34
    risk factors for (Q) 27, (A) 34
    signs of (Q) 27, (A) 34; (Q) 32,
      (A) 36
    sites affected by (Q) 29, (A) 35
    staging of (Q) 30, (A) 35
breast lumps (Q) 121, (A) 142–3
    differential diagnosis of (Q) 32,
      (A) 36
    managing (Q) 28, (A) 34; (Q) 29,
      (A) 35
breast pain (Q) 121, (A) 142
breathlessness (Q) 92, (A) 100
Buerger's disease (Q) 40, (A) 45
Buerger's test (Q) 43, (A) 46
buttocks, claudication in (Q) 41, (A) 45

caecal carcinoma (Q) 118, (A) 140
calcium oxalate (Q) 57, (A) 64
calf, swollen (Q) 42, (A) 46
carbimazole (Q) 126, (A) 148
cardiac tamponade (Q) 96, (A) 101
carotid artery stenosis (Q) 42, (A) 46
carotid endarterectomy (Q) 42, (A) 46
carpal tunnel syndrome (Q) 69,
    (A) 74; (Q) 73, (A) 76
chest drainage (Q) 98, (A) 102
chest injury
    blunt (Q) 97, (A) 101
    penetrating (Q) 96, (A) 101
chest X-ray
    erect (Q) 94, (A) 100
    and ingested bodies (Q) 79, (A) 81
    and neck lumps (Q) 84, (A) 87
cholangiocarcinoma (Q) 23, (A) 26
cholangitis, ascending (Q) 21, (A) 26
cholecystitis (Q) 112, (A) 134;
    (Q) 125, (A) 148
    acute (Q) 19–20, (A) 25

cholestasis, extrahepatic (Q) 20,
    (A) 25
claudication, intermittent (Q) 41,
    (A) 45; (Q) 43, (A) 46
clavicular fracture (Q) 71, (A) 75
Clonorchis sinensis (Q) 23, (A) 26
closed thoracostomy tube drainage
    (Q) 110, (A) 131–2
Clostridium welchii (Q) 95, (A) 100
clotting factors (Q) 84, (A) 87
coins, ingesting (Q) 79, (A) 81
Colles' fracture (Q) 71, (A) 75
colon, transverse (Q) 5, (A) 13
colorectal tumours (Q) 10, (A) 16;
    (Q) 105, (A) 127
constipation (Q) 114, (A) 134–5
    absolute (Q) 6, (A) 13; (Q) 50, (A) 55
Courvoisier's law (Q) 18, (A) 24
cranial nerve palsy (Q) 80, (A) 82
cricothyroidotomy (Q) 89, (A) 99
Crohn's disease (Q) 111, (A) 132
    complications of (Q) 5, (A) 13
    exacerbations of (Q) 18, (A) 24
CT scan, of the head (Q) 90, (A) 99

deep vein thrombosis (Q) 42, (A) 46;
    (Q) 123, (A) 144
detrusor hyperactivity (Q) 63, (A) 66
diabetic neuropathy (Q) 122, (A) 143
diaphragmatic hernia, traumatic
    (Q) 110, (A) 132
diarrhoea (Q) 105, (A) 127; (Q) 111,
    (A) 132
    bloody (Q) 114, (A) 135
    infective (Q) 113, (A) 134
distal fragment (Q) 71, (A) 75
diverticular disease (Q) 117, (A) 138
diverticulitis (Q) 22, (A) 26; (Q) 114,
    (A) 134; (Q) 125, (A) 147
diverticulum perforation (Q) 11,
    (A) 16
duct ectasia (Q) 31, (A) 36
duct papilloma (Q) 30, (A) 35
ductal carcinoma
    invasive (Q) 30–1, (A) 35
    in situ (Q) 28, (A) 34

duodenal ulcer (Q) 11, *(A) 16*
dyspepsia, managing (Q) 4, *(A) 12*
dysphagia (Q) 107, *(A) 128*; (Q) 126,
  (A) 149
    investigations into (Q) 7, *(A) 14*
    managing (Q) 6, *(A) 13*; (Q) 9,
      (A) 15
dysuria (Q) 124, *(A) 146*

ejaculation, retrograde (Q) 59, *(A) 65*
emergency burr hole (Q) 91, *(A) 99*
endoscopic retrograde
  cholangiopancreatography
  (Q) 20–1, *(A) 25*
endoscopy, and dyspepsia (Q) 4,
  (A) 12
epididymo-orchitis (Q) 60, *(A) 65*;
  (Q) 119, *(A) 141*
epigastric pain (Q) 93–4, *(A) 100*;
  (Q) 96, *(A) 101*; (Q) 108, *(A) 129*;
  (Q) 112, *(A) 133–4*; (Q) 114,
  (A) 134; (Q) 125, *(A) 147*
epiglottitis (Q) 78–9, *(A) 81*
erythema multiforme (Q) 5, *(A) 13*
extradural haemorrhage (Q) 91,
  (A) 99

facial droop, unilateral (Q) 80, *(A) 82*
fat necrosis (Q) 32, *(A) 36*; (Q) 121,
  (A) 143
feet
    cold (Q) 38, *(A) 44*
    ischaemic (Q) 41, *(A) 45*
    and peripheral arterial disease
      (Q) 37, *(A) 44*
femoral artery
    embolus in (Q) 42, *(A) 46*
    structures medial to (Q) 47,
      (A) 54
femoral canal (Q) 51, *(A) 55*
    lumps in (Q) 49, *(A) 55*
femoral hernia (Q) 48, *(A) 54*; (Q) 50,
  (A) 55
    strangulated (Q) 53, *(A) 56*;
      (Q) 116, *(A) 137*
femoral neck fracture (Q) 72, *(A) 75*

fibroadenoma (Q) 27, *(A) 34*; (Q) 121,
  (A) 142
fine needle biopsy (Q) 85, *(A) 87*
flail segment (Q) 97, *(A) 101*
flexor digitorum profundus tendon
  (Q) 110, *(A) 131*
fluid challenge (Q) 98, *(A) 102*
fundoplication (Q) 47, *(A) 54*

gallbladder carcinoma (Q) 20, *(A) 25*
gallstones
    and jaundice (Q) 18, *(A) 24*;
      (Q) 20, *(A) 25*
    management of (Q) 19, *(A) 25*
Garden's classification (Q) 72, *(A) 75*
gas embolisation (Q) 49, *(A) 54*
gas gangrene (Q) 95, *(A) 100*
gastric ulcer (Q) 111, *(A) 132*
gastroenteritis (Q) 39, *(A) 44*
gastrografin swallow (Q) 7, *(A) 14*
gastroscopy (Q) 112, *(A) 133*
glandular fever (Q) 108, *(A) 129*
Glasgow Coma Scale (Q) 120, *(A) 141*
goitre (Q) 126, *(A) 149*
groin lumps (Q) 48–9, *(A) 54–5*;
  (Q) 116, *(A) 137*
gynaecomastia (Q) 28, *(A) 34*

haematemesis (Q) 17, *(A) 24*; (Q) 22,
  (A) 26; (Q) 98, *(A) 101*; (Q) 108,
  (A) 130
haematoma, and mastectomy (Q) 31,
  (A) 35
haematuria (Q) 57, *(A) 64*
haemorrhoids (Q) 115, *(A) 135*;
  (Q) 117, *(A) 138*
hallux valgus (Q) 71, *(A) 75*
hand, wasting of intrinsic muscles
  (Q) 73, *(A) 76*
Hartmann's procedure (Q) 11, *(A) 16*
head trauma (Q) 91, *(A) 99*
headache (Q) 90–1, *(A) 99*
height, losing (Q) 69, *(A) 75*
Heller's cardiomyotomy (Q) 3, *(A) 12*
hemicolectomy, left (Q) 8, *(A) 14*
heparin (Q) 123, *(A) 144–5*

hernia, predisposition to (Q) 51,
(A) 55
hernia repair, open (Q) 49, (A) 54
heterophile antibody test (Q) 126,
(A) 148
hiatus hernia (Q) 47, (A) 54
hormonal therapy (Q) 60, (A) 65
humerus, supracondylar fracture of
(Q) 109, (A) 131
hydrocoele (Q) 60–1, (A) 65
hyperthyroidism (Q) 126, (A) 148
hypotension, and catheterisation
(Q) 63, (A) 66

idiopathic thrombocytopaenia
(Q) 115, (A) 136
ilioinguinal nerve (Q) 52, (A) 55;
(Q) 90, (A) 99
immunoglobulin, intravenous
(Q) 115, (A) 136
incisional hernia (Q) 52, (A) 56;
(Q) 118, (A) 139
incontinence (Q) 124, (A) 146
inferior epigastric vessels (Q) 51,
(A) 55
inflammatory bowel disease (Q) 105,
(A) 127
inguinal canal (Q) 52, (A) 55
inguinal hernia (Q) 116, (A) 136
    causes of (Q) 47, (A) 54
    direct (Q) 51, (A) 55; (Q) 90,
    (A) 99
    hot (Q) 50, (A) 55
    indirect (Q) 48, (A) 54; (Q) 51,
    (A) 55; (Q) 119, (A) 140
intervertebral disc collapse (Q) 68, (A) 74
intestinal obstruction, presentation of
(Q) 9, (A) 15
intussusception (Q) 8, (A) 15
involution (Q) 121, (A) 142
iron replacement (Q) 9, (A) 15
irritable bowel syndrome (Q) 112,
(A) 133–4
ischaemic colitis (Q) 105, (A) 127–8
ischaemic heart disease (Q) 122,
(A) 143

ischaemic limbs (Q) 41, (A) 45;
(Q) 110, (A) 132

jaundice
    investigations for (Q) 20, (A) 25;
    (Q) 22, (A) 26
    painless (Q) 18, (A) 24
jaw swelling (Q) 126, (A) 148
joint aspiration (Q) 67, (A) 74
joint cast (Q) 70, (A) 75

knee, swollen (Q) 67–8, (A) 74
koilonychia (Q) 3, (A) 12

laparoscopic cholecystectomy (Q) 21,
(A) 26; (Q) 23, (A) 26
laparoscopy, diagnostic (Q) 125,
(A) 147
laparotomy scar (Q) 114, (A) 134–5
large bowel obstructions (Q) 21,
(A) 26
laryngeal mask airway (Q) 120,
(A) 141
laryngomalacia (Q) 78, (A) 81
left iliac fossa pain (Q) 125, (A) 147
leg and foot ulcers (Q) 122, (A) 143
leg pain (Q) 68, (A) 74; (Q) 123,
(A) 144
legs
    cold (Q) 41, (A) 45
    complications of fracture fixation
    (Q) 94, (A) 100
    deformed (Q) 73, (A) 76
Leriche's syndrome (Q) 41, (A) 45
Littré's hernia (Q) 50, (A) 55
lymph glands, submandibular (Q) 126,
(A) 148
lymph nodes (Q) 83, (A) 87
    reactive (Q) 116, (A) 137
lymphadenopathy
    in lower limb (Q) 122, (A) 143
    secondary (Q) 107, (A) 128
lymphoma (Q) 116, (A) 137

Mallory–Weiss tear (Q) 4, (A) 12;
(Q) 111, (A) 132

March fracture (Q) 109, *(A) 131*
mastectomy, complications from
(Q) 31, *(A) 35*
mastitis
    acute (Q) 121, *(A) 142*
    periductal (Q) 29, *(A) 35*
Maydl's hernia (Q) 52, *(A) 56*
Meckel's diverticulum (Q) 8, *(A) 15*;
    (Q) 111, *(A) 133*
medullary carcinoma (Q) 85, *(A) 87*
melaena (Q) 9, *(A) 15*
mesentery (Q) 10, *(A) 16*
metaplasia (Q) 5, *(A) 13*
microcalcifications (Q) 33, *(A) 36*
mononucleosis (Q) 126, *(A) 148*
multiple sclerosis (Q) 59, *(A) 64*
mumps (Q) 79, *(A) 82*; (Q) 107,
    (A) 128; (Q) 119, *(A) 141*
Murphy's sign (Q) 18, *(A) 24*
muscular strain (Q) 123, *(A) 144*

nasogastric tube (Q) 125, *(A) 147*
neck lumps (Q) 83–5, *(A) 87*; (Q) 107,
    (A) 128
neck swelling (Q) 126, *(A) 148*
neck wounds (Q) 110, *(A) 131*
neck X-ray (Q) 86, *(A) 88*
neoplasia, and bowel obstruction
    (Q) 8, *(A) 14*
nephritis, chronic interstitial (Q) 62,
    (A) 66
neuropathic ulcers (Q) 122, *(A) 143*
night splints (Q) 69, *(A) 74*
nipple discharge (Q) 30, *(A) 35*
    bloody (Q) 121, *(A) 142*
    cheesy (Q) 31–2, *(A) 36*
nipple retraction (Q) 29, *(A) 35*;
    (Q) 31–2, *(A) 36*
nosebleed (Q) 84, *(A) 87*
NSAIDs (non-steroidal anti-
    inflammatory drugs) (Q) 111,
    (A) 132; (Q) 123, *(A) 144*

obturator hernia (Q) 49, *(A) 55*
oesophageal cancer (Q) 4, *(A) 12*;
    (Q) 111, *(A) 132–3*

oesophageal perforation (Q) 7, *(A) 14*
oesophageal varices (Q) 108, *(A) 130*
oesophagus
    foreign bodies in (Q) 79, *(A) 81*
    replacement of (Q) 5, *(A) 13*
Ogilvie's syndrome (Q) 125, *(A) 147*
open reduction (Q) 72, *(A) 75*;
    (Q) 94, *(A) 100*
orchitis (Q) 119, *(A) 141*
osteoarthritis (Q) 123, *(A) 144*
osteoporosis (Q) 69, *(A) 75*; (Q) 73,
    (A) 76
osteosclerotic metastases (Q) 58,
    (A) 64
oxygen facemask (Q) 120, *(A) 141*

Paget's disease (Q) 73, *(A) 76*
pancreatic cancer (Q) 19, *(A) 25*
pancreatic pseudocyst (Q) 108,
    (A) 129
pancreatitis, acute (Q) 17–18, *(A) 24*;
    (Q) 125, *(A) 147*
paralytic ileus (Q) 23, *(A) 26*
parotid gland (Q) 79, *(A) 82*
Pemberton's sign (Q) 86, *(A) 88*
peptic ulcer, perforated (Q) 93–4,
    (A) 100; (Q) 114, *(A) 134*
pericardiocentesis (Q) 96, *(A) 101*
peripheral arterial disease (Q) 37,
    (A) 44
peripheral vascular disease (Q) 43,
    (A) 46
pharyngeal pouch (Q) 107, *(A) 128*
pleomorphic adenomas (Q) 80,
    (A) 82
Plummer–Vinson syndrome (Q) 3,
    (A) 12; (Q) 9, *(A) 15*
proctocolectomy, restorative (Q) 10,
    (A) 15
prostate, transurethral resection of
    (Q) 59, *(A) 65*
prostate cancer (Q) 124, *(A) 145–6*
    metastases of (Q) 58, *(A) 64*;
    (Q) 60, *(A) 65*
prostatitis (Q) 124, *(A) 146*
pruritus ani (Q) 117, *(A) 138*

pulmonary embolism (Q) 123,
(A) 144–5
pyloric stenosis (Q) 9, (A) 15
pyoderma gangrenosum (Q) 122,
(A) 144

radionuclide scan (Q) 62, (A) 66
Ramstedt's pyloromyotomy (Q) 9,
(A) 15
rebound tenderness (Q) 11, (A) 16
rectal bleeding (Q) 111, (A) 133;
(Q) 115, (A) 136
rectal carcinoma (Q) 10, (A) 16;
(Q) 115, (A) 136; (Q) 117, (A) 138
rectal pain (Q) 124, (A) 146
recti, divarication of (Q) 108, (A) 129
rectus sheath haematoma (Q) 118,
(A) 139
renal tract calculi (Q) 57, (A) 64
respiration, paradoxical (Q) 97,
(A) 101
rest pain (Q) 43, (A) 46
Richter's hernia (Q) 49, (A) 55
right iliac fossa
    pain (Q) 118, (A) 140; (Q) 125,
    (A) 147
    tenderness (Q) 22, (A) 26;
    (Q) 114, (A) 135
right upper quadrant pain (Q) 125,
(A) 148
road traffic accidents (Q) 89, (A) 99;
(Q) 110, (A) 131–2
Rockall score (Q) 98, (A) 101

salivary duct, blocked (Q) 126,
(A) 148
saphenofemoral incompetence (Q) 38,
(A) 44
saphenous system, long (Q) 38,
(A) 44
scaphoid fracture (Q) 70, (A) 75;
(Q) 73, (A) 76; (Q) 109, (A) 131
scapula, winged (Q) 68, (A) 74
scrotal support (Q) 61, (A) 65
scrotum, swollen (Q) 62, (A) 65–6;
(Q) 107, (A) 128; (Q) 119, (A) 140–1

seizures (Q) 109, (A) 130; (Q) 120,
(A) 141
seminoma (Q) 119, (A) 140
Sengstaken–Blakemore tube (Q) 22,
(A) 26
serratus anterior (Q) 68, (A) 74
serum amylase (Q) 114, (A) 134;
(Q) 125, (A) 147
sexual impotence (Q) 41, (A) 45
shoulder dislocations (Q) 109, (A) 130
sialogram (Q) 126, (A) 148
slurred speech (Q) 37, (A) 44
small bowel obstruction (Q) 114,
(A) 134–5; (Q) 118, (A) 140
smoking (Q) 27, (A) 34
    and Buerger's disease (Q) 40,
    (A) 45
sphincterotomy (Q) 21, (A) 25
splenic flexure, cancer at (Q) 8, (A) 14
splenic rupture (Q) 108, (A) 129
squamous cell carcinoma (Q) 4,
(A) 12; (Q) 122, (A) 143
stab wounds (Q) 90, (A) 99; (Q) 110,
(A) 131–2
stereotactic biopsy (Q) 33, (A) 36
steroids
    complications of (Q) 20, (A) 25
    and immunosuppression (Q) 67,
    (A) 74
    and ulcerative colitis (Q) 115,
    (A) 136
stridor, acquired paediatric (Q) 78,
(A) 81
subarachnoid haemorrhage (Q) 90,
(A) 99
subclavian artery (Q) 71, (A) 75
subdural haematoma (Q) 95, (A) 101
sutures, removing (Q) 92, (A) 100
swallowing, difficulty in (Q) 3, (A) 12
synovial fluid aspirate (Q) 70, (A) 75

Takayasu's arteritis (Q) 41, (A) 46
technetium thyroid scan (Q) 126,
(A) 148
tension pneumothorax (Q) 92–3,
(A) 100; (Q) 110, (A) 131–2

testicles
    swollen (Q) 60–1, *(A) 65*
    undescended (Q) 61, *(A) 65*
testicular lump (Q) 61, *(A) 65*
testicular torsion (Q) 62, *(A) 65–6*;
    (Q) 97, *(A) 101*; (Q) 119, *(A) 140*
thenar eminence (Q) 84, *(A) 87*
thoracic inlet obstruction (Q) 86,
    (A) 88
thoracic outlet syndrome (Q) 84,
    (A) 87
thoracotomy (Q) 98, *(A) 102*
thrombolysis, interoperative (Q) 42,
    (A) 46
thyroglossal cyst (Q) 107, *(A) 128–9*
thyroid cancer (Q) 85, *(A) 87*;
    (Q) 126, *(A) 148*
thyroidectomy, complications of
    (Q) 85, *(A) 87*; (Q) 92, *(A) 100*
thyroiditis (Q) 107, *(A) 128*
tibial fracture, spiral (Q) 109,
    (A) 130–1
tidal volume (Q) 97, *(A) 101*
toe, swollen (Q) 70, *(A) 75*
toe pain (Q) 109, *(A) 131*
tonsillectomy (Q) 78, *(A) 81*
tonsillitis, acute (Q) 77, *(A) 81*
total parenteral nutrition (Q) 6, *(A) 13*
trachea, deviated (Q) 92–3, *(A) 100*
tracheal intubation (Q) 120, *(A) 141–2*
trusses (Q) 50, *(A) 55*
twisting injury (Q) 109, *(A) 130–1*

ulcerative colitis (Q) 6, *(A) 13–14*;
    (Q) 10, *(A) 15*; (Q) 114, *(A) 135*;
    (Q) 117, *(A) 137–8*

acute attack (Q) 115, *(A) 136*
and ulcers (Q) 122, *(A) 144*
ultrasound
    abdominal (Q) 21, *(A) 26*;
        (Q) 112, *(A) 133–4*
    of breasts (Q) 28, *(A) 34*
    and deep vein thrombosis (Q) 42,
        (A) 46
    and gallstones (Q) 125, *(A) 148*
    of the neck (Q) 37, *(A) 44*
    scrotal (Q) 61, *(A) 65*
urethral catheterisation (Q) 58,
    (A) 64
urgency, urinary (Q) 58, *(A) 64*
urinary catheterisation (Q) 62–3,
    (A) 66
urinary infection, recurrent (Q) 124,
    (A) 146

varicose veins (Q) 38–9, *(A) 44–5*
varicosities, complications of (Q) 39,
    (A) 45
venous insufficiency (Q) 40, *(A) 45*
vesicoureteric calculus (Q) 57,
    (A) 64
vomiting
    and bowel obstructions (Q) 114,
        (A) 135
    projectile (Q) 9, *(A) 15*

warfarin (Q) 123, *(A) 144–5*
weight loss, unintentional (Q) 112,
    (A) 133; (Q) 117, *(A) 138*
Whipple's procedure (Q) 19,
    (A) 25
wrist lacerations (Q) 95, *(A) 100*

CPD with Radcliffe

You can now use a selection of our books to achieve CPD (Continuing Professional Development) points through directed reading.

We provide a free online form and downloadable certificate for your appraisal portfolio. Look for the CPD logo and register with us at: www.radcliffehealth.com/cpd

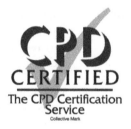